The Greatest Hits of

HEALTH TIPS

the most commonly asked questions for the radio health expert

by
Dr. Patrick Quillin

published by
Nutrition Times Press, Inc.
Tulsa, OK

📖 **Other books by Dr. Patrick Quillin**

La Costa Prescription for Longer Life, Fawcett Crest, NY, 1985
Healing Nutrients, Random House, NY, 1987
La Costa Book of Nutrition, World Almanac, NY, 1988
Safe Eating, Evans, NY, 1990
Adjuvant Nutrition in Cancer Treatment, CTRF, Arlington Hts, IL, 1993
Amish Folk Medicine, Leader Company, N. Canton, OH, 1993
Beating Cancer with Nutrition, Nutrition Times Press, Tulsa, 1994
Wisdom & Healing Power of Whole Foods, Vitamix, Cleveland, 1994
Healing Secrets from the Bible, Nutrition Times Press, Tulsa, 1996
Honey, Garlic & Vinegar, Leader Co., North Canton, OH, 1996

TO ORDER Dr. Quillin's books, SEE YOUR BOOKSTORE or HEALTH FOOD STORE OR CALL 1-800-444-2524

copyright 1996 Patrick Quillin
ISBN 0-9638372-2-2

Printed in the United States of America

Quantity discounts are available from:
Nutrition Times Press, Inc.
Box 700512
Tulsa, OK 74170
phone & fax 918-495-1137

On your letterhead, include information concerning the intended use of the books and the number of books you wish to purchase.

DEDICATION

To Richard J Stephenson,
    For your uncommon valor and intelligence in moving the American health care system in a more rational direction.

ACKNOWLEDGEMENTS

    Many thanks to all the fine people at the Oasis Network who have been so supportive of Health Tips.

IMPORTANT NOTICE

HOW THIS ALL GOT STARTED

☞ "The doctor of the future will give no medicine, but will involve the patient in the proper use of food, fresh air, and exercise." Thomas Edison, American inventor

In the later part of 1991, I spent time with David Warren of the Oasis Christian Radio Network, discussing subjects of mutual interest. We developed the concept of recording a series of one minute radio spots, or public service announcements, to be broadcast during the morning and evening rush hour. The title would be Health Tips. The content would be short and pithey answers to the questions that are commonly asked of me. There have been 8 "batches" to date of Health Tips, which provides the breaks for the 8 chapters in this book.

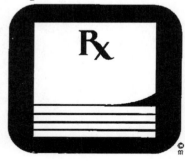

We wanted to make this one minute radio spot a very relevant and palatable moment to bring healthy thoughts to the American public. You see, we have a serious problem in this country. We are on the verge of a "health care meltdown". In spite of spending over $1 trillion per year in health care and having the world's most productive farmers to fill our grocery stores,

Americans still have among the world's highest rates for heart disease, cancer, diabetes, Alzheimer's, osteoporosis, arthritis, and infant mortality. Clearly, we cannot buy health, but must earn it. We build the foundations for health and disease resistance through a good diet, exercise, toxin avoidance, supplements, good attitude, sunshine, rest, fresh air, and a close relationship with God.

Oftentimes the American health care system spends lavishly and wastefully on our sick people. Drugs can cost $1000 per day. Hospitalization can cost more than $3000 per day. Sophisticated medical equipment, like CAT scans and MRI (magnetic resonance imaging), can cost millions of dollars to purchase. And yet, amidst this impressive array of high tech equipment and drugs, we somehow forget the obvious: the need to nourish the body, mind, and spirit.

HEALTH TIPS are an accumulation of many years of questions from people like you. There are no fancy textbook explanations here. Only practical and easy solutions for common health problems. May you live a long, healthy, exuberant, and joyous life!!

Patrick Quillin, PhD,RD,CNS
Tulsa, Oklahoma

Chapter 1

📖

HEALTH TIPS

☞ "Each patient carries his own "doctor" inside him. We are at our best when we give the doctor who resides within a chance to go to work." Albert Schweitzer, MD, medical missionary

(opening) This is Health Tips and I'm Dr. Patrick Quillin. Today's question comes from ___.
(closing) God bless and good health.

-physical risks in obesity

TN of Broken Arrow. I have been fighting the battle of the bulge for years and have about given up. My grandmother used to say that fat people lived longer. Why should I lose weight?

Thank you TN. In your grandmother's day, overweight people were less likely to get

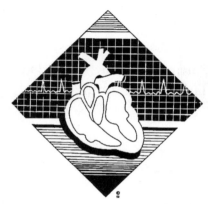

tuberculosis, which was a major killer at the turn of the century. Today, obesity is nearly equal to cigarette smoking as a risk factor for major crippling and fatal diseases. Overweight people are more likely to suffer diabetes, heart disease, stroke, arthritis, cancer (especially of the breast), and even accidents. You have many good reasons to shed that excess poundage.

-emotional risks in obesity

GR of Oolagah. Are overweight people typically as jolly as old Saint Nick?

Thank you GR. Some are, but most are not. Psychology studies find that most overweight people have a low self esteem, and suffer from depression and lethargy more often than people of normal weight. This could be due to our society's obsession with a certain Hollywood image, or it could be from a genuine problem associated with being overweight. Jolly and plump old Saint Nick is, unfortunately, the exception to the rule. All the more reason to make an effort to trim down.

-reasons why most diets fail

CT of Midwest City. I have fought a losing battle for years on my waistline. Why do so many of my efforts fail?

Thanks CT. Obesity experts have found that 95% of unstructured diets will fail in the long run. That's a pretty dismal track record. The reasons cited for failure at weight loss include: expecting someone or something else to do it for you, expecting a cure, and expecting immediate results.

Actually, you must take responsibility for your weight loss, since no one else can life your lifestyle except you. Also, there is no cure for obesity, only lifetime maintenance. And since it takes years to add the weight, it will take months of patience to slowly melt away the unwanted fat. Knowledge is your greatest ally at this point.

-easiest way to permanently lose weight, fat
WT of Oklahoma City. How do the stars in Hollywood manage to stay looking lean and young long after most others their age have gained girth?

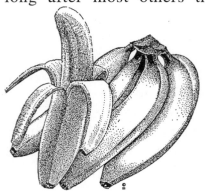

Very good question, WT. Although we see our favorite stars on TV eating and drinking excessively, actually most of them are quite diligent about their fitness program. These people know that their profitable livelihood depends on looking good and so they take good care of themselves. One of the best kept secrets among Hollywood celebrities is the low fat diet. If you do nothing else but eat less fat, you will find it easier to lose weight and maintain that trim figure. This means eating less cheese, pizza, deep fried foods, hot dogs, bologna, hamburgers, and others. The low fat diet works.

-set point theory
DB of Sapulpa. With the best of intentions, I can't seem to break through a certain weight

barrier. At a certain point, the fat sticks to me like velcro. What can I do?

Thanks DB. Scientists at Harvard University found that each of us has a set point, or weight at which our body wants to stay at. This set point is based upon genetics, body fat accumulated in childhood, dietary intake, and exercise. If you are making a genuine effort at eating a decent diet, the only way to break through this set point barrier is to exercise. Regular activity will lower your body's ideal weight, or set point, so that it becomes easy to maintain.

-eating habits, replace them

LT of Shawnee. I drive a truck for a living and snack while driving to ease the long lonely hours on the road. I know I shouldn't eat so much, but I can't stop, even though I've tried to.

Thanks LT. It is much easier to replace an unwanted habit with a good one rather than to just plain stop cold turkey. When your child is drawing on the kitchen wall, it is best to offer him or her a drawing pad of paper as a substitute behavior, rather than just telling them to stop it. Same with your eating habits. You need to replace the unhealthy highway grazing with a healthier habit, such as listening to books on tape, learning a foreign language, chewing gum, or if you must snack, then eat low calorie foods such as fruit, dried fruit, or whole grain breakfast cereals. Happy trails.

-habits of lean people

FP of Tulsa. What habits can I teach my kids so they don't end up with the same weight problem that has been in my family for generations.

Your concern is noble FP, since childhood is where we acquire our eating habits and even excess fat cells from overeating. An overweight child will likely have an uphill battle with obesity for much of their life. You can start some simple procedures for your kids that install healthy eating habits, like small frequent meals, eat a low fat soup before each dinner, chew food at least 25 times per mouthful, use smaller plates to make a little food look like more. Reward your children with something other than food, otherwise they may develop a lifelong bad habit of rewarding themselves with a cheeseburger everytime they feel down. You can start some healthy habits today that will be one of the best gifts that a parent can offer their children: good health.

-genetics & obesity

SP of Okmulgee. My husband and I both have a weight problem and we are worried that our children will end up with the same problem. Are our children at risk?

Thank you SP. Yes, overweight parents often do have overweight children.

Scientists find that if one parent is overweight, the odds of having an overweight child are 40%, while if both parents are overweight, the odds increase to 80%. No doubt some of this risk comes from body type. God created an endless variety of body shapes and sizes. Some people are larger and store fat more efficiently. But the main reason that overweight parents have overweight kids is lifestyle: eating too fast, eating high fat foods, eating when under stress, sedentary habits, and others are all part of the lifestyle that molds children into a pattern that promotes obesity. You cannot change your genetic makeup, but you can change your lifestyle to make your kids healthier.

-value of exercise

CK of Jenks. I just don't seem to have the time or energy for exercise. Is exercise really that important. And how can a busy mom make time in her day for exercise?

Thanks CK. Yes, exercise is really that important. A well respected physician from Stanford University has pointed out that most of the diseases in our society are related to dis-use of the body; meaning no exercise. Exercise lowers the levels of fats in the blood, burns up stores of body fats, purges the body of toxins through sweat, elevates basal metabolism so that you can eat more without gaining weight, reduces stress, and even improves the efficiency of the immune system. Even busy people can find 20 minutes per day for stationery biking, stair climbing, indoor cross country skiing, aerobics with a video tape, or just brisk walking. You will find the rewards well worth the efforts.

-breast cancer & obesity

HJ of Midwest City. I've been reading about all the celebrities with breast cancer, including: former first lady, Mrs. Ford, Jill Ireland, Ann Jillian, and others. What can I do to lower my risk for breast cancer?

Thanks HJ. The risk for breast cancer in American women has escalated from one out of 20 in 1950 to one out of 9 in 1990. While early detection is a key in successful treatment, an even better strategy is to not get cancer. Scientists find that the primary risk factors for cancer include exposure to toxins (such as tobacco, alcohol, drugs, and pollutants), poor diet (which most Americans indulge in), and stress or unhappiness. Of the dietary factors, by increasing your intake of yogurt, fiber, vitamins E, A, C, and selenium, while also lowering your intake of fat, cholesterol, and caffeine, then you will have made major progress toward cutting your cancer risks. Also, overweight is a major risk factor toward breast cancer.

-longer life through ideal nutrition

VE of Tulsa. What are these studies about undernutrition without malnutrition, what does that mean?

Thanks VE. Of all the scientific evidence linking nutrition to health and longevity, the strongest link is between food restriction and long life. Across the board, in both animal and human studies, if you eat less and make that food of high nutrient density, then you are dramatically improving your chances of living a longer and healthier life. This means eating more fruits, vegetables, whole grains, legumes, and clean water, while taking in less fat. Interestingly, Biblical references tell us that Moses lived to be about 120 years, while the latest scientific studies claim that following this regimen of undernutrition without malnutrition will produce a potential lifespan of about 120 years.

-appetite & zinc, other nutrients

AR of Norman. Sometimes I eat even when I am not hungry. What is wrong with my appetite?

Thanks AR. Eating and appetite are complex issues. While most creatures on earth only eat when they are physically hungry and in need of food, humans eat for many more reasons, including stress, need for comfort, boredom, depression, oral fixation, etc. You may need to speak with a counselor about your overeating problem. Alternatively, there are also nutrients which help your body to maintain a healthy appetite, including zinc, folacin, thiamin, and more. Some studies have shown that a malnourished person is more likely to have bizarre eating habits. Perhaps what you need is quality broad spectrum supplement to fill in the nutritional gaps in your diet. Your overeating problems may diminish once your body has the nutrients that it needs.

-fiber, Graham crackers, roughage

JY of Oklahoma City. I need to lose weight, but don't like the feeling of having an empty stomach all the time. What can I do?

Thanks JY. One of the miracle nutrients of the 90s is fiber. Although fiber has been in our food supply since the beginning of time, it was in the 1950s that food technologists figured out how to remove fiber from our foods. With that tragic loss came a wave of heart disease, obesity, diabetes, 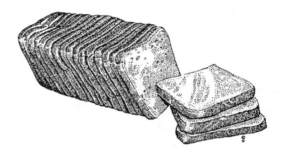 and cancer. We now know why God put fiber in the food supply. Even though fiber is indigestible, it is highly essential for adding non-caloric bulk to our food intake. With a high fiber diet, which is found only in plant food, you do not have to experience hunger while losing weight.

-dangers of fasting

OT of Claremore. My husband says that the best diet is to just stop eating. Is fasting a good idea?

Thanks OT. Short term fasting, such as one day per week, for healthy people may be a good idea. However, long term fasting is not a good idea. Over a decade ago, 16 people died on what was appropriately titled the last chance diet. These people died from lean tissue wasting, since their body was not getting enough protein stores, and also from electrolyte imbalances. Long term fasting not only lowers your basal metabolism to make you a more efficient machine for storing calories as fat, but it also challenges the body to draw on its nutrients reserves. In the typical American who is living on junk food and fast food, there are no nutrient reserves. Make sure that you get enough protein while in your weight loss phase.

-fat burning nutrients

TC of Sand Springs. Since we have opened up the human gene and gone to the moon, do we know of any nutrients that can make weight loss a little easier and safer?

Thanks TC. You are right, there is a way of using the latest in nutritional science to make weight loss safer and quicker. Carnitine is a nutrient that is essential for the body to burn fat. Vitamin C is a nutrient that helps to regulate the dumping of fats and cholesterol into the bloodstream. Chromium is a mineral that is crucial for the efficient burning of sugar in the body cells. Vitamin E is vital for preventing the "rusting" of fats in the body. The typical American is low in these "fat processing" nutrients and could use some supplementation to make their weight reduction program faster, more efficient, safer, and without hunger pangs.

Chapter 2

📖

HEALTH TIPS

☞ "There can never be any real opposition between religion and science, for the one is the complement of the other. Every advance in knowledge brings us face to face with the mystery of our own being." Max Planck, famous scientist

(opening) This is Health Tips and I'm Dr. Patrick Quillin. Today's question comes from___.
(closing) God Bless and good health.

-thyroid

TN of Broken Arrow. I've had weight problems all my life. My momma used to take thyroid pills. Do you think low thyroid could be part of my weight problems?

Thank you TN. While most of us have adequate thyroid output to survive, experts estimate that about 40% of the population suffers

from chronic low thyroid production, which surfaces as easy weight gain, hypoglycemia, coldness, constipation, reproductive problems in women, lethargy, and even anxiety in some people. If your temperature first thing in the morning is less than 98.2 degrees F. then you need to talk to your doctor about getting desicated thyroid supplements. Read one of the books by Drs. Langer or Barnes about thyroid. It is the master gland in the body and regulates all functions.

-juicing

RG of Midwest City. I saw this guy on TV talk about juicing as the magical way to cure anything you got. What do you think about juicing?

Thank you RG. I have often emphasized the importance of eating more fruits and vegetables. By juicing fruits and vegetables, you can consume more of some of the precious nutrients that encourage good health, including indoles from cabbage, ellagic acid from apples, and carotenoids from carrots. However, don't juice instead of eating the whole plant. There is good evidence that plant food is a delicately woven tapestry of important ingredients, some of which are lost in juicing. My wife and I juice, then use the leftover pulp to make a delicious cake, like carrot cake. Also, make sure that you consume your fruit and vegetable juices along with a meal, since the sugar content of the juice can elevate blood glucose and insulin levels and create problems in prostaglandins. Juicing is no cure all, by any means, but when done right it is a valuable way to get more nutrients in the diet.

-magnesium & heart disease

CT of Owasso. My doctor has put me on all kinds of medication and I keep waking up in the night with muscle cramps. What can I do?

Thank you CT. Many medications can cause a loss of potassium and magnesium from the body, which can express itself as muscle cramps, fatigue, irritability, and even heart problems such as cardiac arrest. In the rare instances when young healthy athletes die while exercising, many experts feel that an electrolyte imbalance is the cause. You can get more potassium from plant food, especially apricots, bananas, and cantaloupe. Magnesium is a bit more difficult to get in the diet, being found in soybeans, shrimp, wheat germ, molasses, spinach, oysters, and peas. Both minerals are crucial for nerve and muscle function. You may even want to consider using potassium chloride, or salt substitute, as a way of supplementing your potassium intake.

-why is there more emphasis on drugs than nutrients

TW of Oklahoma City. I read the paper all the time and see all the money that government and industry spends researching drugs. Why don't people spend more money on researching vitamins and natural things that don't have all those side effects?

Thank you TW. Long ago, the government decided that natural substances, like vitamins, could not be patented. Without the protection of a patent, big business is hesitant to spend any money on promotion and marketing. Hence, we have created an unhealthy atmosphere for research in this country. We need to allow scientists to research and develop the most effective agents possible to fight disease, not just develop the most patentable substances, which is where we are at now. Unfortunately, much research money is wasted trying to find a synthetic derivative of 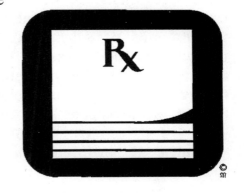 an effective natural agent, merely for the means of profitabillity. Maybe our listeners can figure out a solution to this stigma of researching natural non-toxic products for health care.

-most toxic of nutrients; for supplement caution

KO of Sapulpa. I've been learning a lot from your health tips. Sometimes you tell us to take vitamins in reasonable amounts. What is a reasonable and what is a toxic level of vitamins.

thanks KO. While a well designed supplement can add measurably to one's nutrient intake and long term health outlook, there are a few nutrients that merit attention for their possible toxicity.

Selenium, vitamin A, and vitamin D are the most likely to create a problem if taken in excess. Another hazard is when children swallow an entire bottle of vitamins that are enriched with iron, since iron toxicity in children can be dangerous. Scientists feel that toxicity of selenium starts at about 2000 micrograms daily for months which is far above what you need for health, vitamin A could be toxic in pregnant women in as little as 25,000 units per day, and vitamin D intake should not exceed 1000 units daily without a doctor's monitoring. While nutrient supplements are relatively safe and beneficial, they still should be treated with respect and intelligence.

-vitamin C supplements & longer life

KW of Tulsa. Is there any evidence that taking extra vitamin C will help prevent anything.

Thanks KW. One of the original promoters of higher than normal vitamin C intake was Professor Linus Pauling, twice nobel laureate, who has since outlived most of his critics and is 92 this year. there is scientific research showing that women who consume less than 90 milligrams daily of vitamin C are at higher risk for ovarian cancer. A recent report from the University of California shows that men who take vitamin C supplements of 500 milligrams daily can expect to add roughly 6 years to their lives. Other studies have found a link between chronic low intake of vitamin C and kidney stones, heart disease, cancer, and gum problems. I encourage people to consume at least 500 mg from

a diet high in fresh fruits and vegetables and/or
supplements.

-new health programs from the government

AJ of Shawnee. I keep hearing these
politicians talking about what they are going to do
for our country's health problems. Do you see any
good ideas out there.

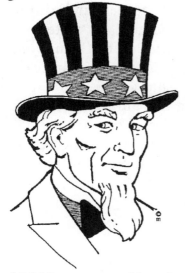

Thanks AJ. Our nation
now spends 12% of our gross
national product, or over
$800 billion per year on
sickness care, not health care.
We spend about 1% of that
money on health care or
preventive measures. While
a number of policitians have
created complex and usually
quite costly solutions to our
sickness dilemma, they are
all missing a critical element:
prevention. It costs about
$2000 to provide decent nourishment and medical
care for a pregnant women, but it costs over $1
million if her baby is defective and left for the
government to tend. The same ratio applies to
cancer, heart disease, mental illness, and our other
illnesses. Somehow we have forgotten that
valuable expression "an ounce of prevention is
worth a pound of cure". We now realize that most
diseases are difficult at best to treat and far easier
and cheaper to prevent.

-summertime & cool snacks for kids

KT of Sand Springs. My kids and all the neighbor kids are home for the summer and spending it in my kitchen. What drinks and snacks can I make them that will be good for them and cheap for me to fix.

Good thought KT. A tasty, cheap, and nutritious beverage is to take unsweetened fruit juice (preferably orange, grape, or apple) and dilute it with twice the recommended amount of water, then add 1 teaspoon of powdered vitamin C and one teaspoon of potassium chloride (or salt substitute) per quart of fluid. For a great snack,quarter then peel fresh oranges and put them in the freezer. take out a frozen orange section for a popsickle. Cools them down while nourishing them. Also, pour fruit flavored yogurt into popsickle molds and let them freeze. Also, try barbecuing turkey hot dogs, which have considerably less fat. Have a great summer.

-milk allergy & childhood earaches

JJ of Jenks. My young boy has been having earaches for the last few years. The doctors medication gets through with one earache and my boy starts on another earache. What's wrong?

Thanks JJ. Your son may be suffering from allergies. Milk is the most common allergen in the world, with more than 20% of people allergic to milk protein and up to 60% unable to digest milk sugar. Allergies can cause an inflammation of the mucous membranes in the upper respiratory tract, which seals off the eustachian tube that leads to the ear, which creates an excellent environment for infections. Try taking your son off of dairy products for at least one week. No cheese, ice cream, milk, butter, margarine, or sour cream. it takes some effort, but may clear up a problem that cannot be cured with drugs.

-tamoxifen & taxol as cancer treatments
BW of Norman. I've read of tamoxifen and taxol as new wonder drugs against cancer. But I've heard that before. Do you think we will ever develop a wonder drug against cancer?

Thought provoking question BW. Only time will tell and I am optimistic about our efforts in cancer research. However, cancer is such a multi-faceted disease with almost limitless causes that a wonder pill against all cancer is unlikely. More likely there will be various drugs, techniques, psychological methods, and nutritional programs developed which will mesh together like gears in a finely crafted automobile. Synergism, or the sum being greater than the individual parts, is the key word in cancer therapy today. By eliminating the causes of the cancer and stimulating the patient's own internal healing abilities while concurrently providing aggressive medical therapy to reduce tumor burden, we are well en route today toward helping more cancer patients than ever before.

-risk factors of osteoporosis
TB of Bixby. Both my grandmothers got osteoporosis in their later years and died in the

hospital of complications. What is osteoporosis and can I prevent it?

Excellent forethought TB. Osteoporosis is a hollowing of the bones, or demineralization which is most common in post-menopausal women and alcoholics. There are many factors that contribute to this long term drain on bone stores, including cigarettes, alcohol, caffeine, stress, sedentary lifestyle, too much protein and phosphorus, too little calcium, magnesium, and vitamin D. Some new data even shows that a mere 1 milligram per day of vitamin K will help stop the loss of bone minerals that leads to osteoporosis. Preventing this disease is a matter of general lifestyle changes rather than just taking antacids for a calcium supply.

-FDA & nutrients

TQ of Okmulgee. I read in the paper that the Texas State Department of Health seized a supply of Coenzyme Q in health food stores. What is this stuff and why would the health dept. take something out of a health food store?

Timely question TQ. The government has maintained a position for the last 60 years that if a product has therapeutic value then it must be under the control of the Food and Drug Administration and be available by prescription only. The whole nutrition story has created a serious dilemma for the government. Nutrients do have therapeutic action when used properly and rarely have any side effects since they are extracted from food stuffs. Hence, nutrients like

Coenzyme Q sit precariously in a baffling new zone for FDA regulation. CoQ has been shown in many well conducted university studies to help heart disease patients. While CoQ has no toxicity, the government has been indecisive about what to do regarding the therapeutic value of CoQ.

-vitamin D & psoriasis

MN of Bartlesville. My daughter has been having problems with a skin rash that just won't go away, even with medication. Can you suggest anything?

Thanks MN. Skin problems can be an indication of allergies, both food and inhalant type; or may indicate a fatty acid problem such as from too much saturated and hydrogenated fats and not enough essential fatty acids. Since the skin is considered a sacrificial organ, many malnutritive conditions will surface in skin problems, including vitamin A and zinc deficiencies. Skin problems are also linked to emotional upset. However, a new vitamin D skin lotion has shown great effectiveness against many drug resistant forms of psoriasis and eczema. Talk with your dermatologist about this new vitamin D ointment.

-nutrients reverse pre-malignant conditions

CG of Wagoner. My dad has been diagnosed as having oral leukoplakia, I guess from all the pipe smoking he does. What's next?

Thanks CG. Oral leukoplakia is a pre-malignant condition, meaning that it is not active spreading cancer yet, but it is too close for comfort.

It usually shows up as a whitish film in the mouth that cannot be scraped off and is most common in smokers and chewers. Fortunately, some new evidence shows that high doses of vitamin A under a doctor's care can reverse this condition. It is best to stop the tobacco use while on this therapy. Don't wait until the condition becomes full blown mouth cancer.

-Time Magazine article on "power of vitamins"

FI of Claremore. There was an article in Time magazine recently that said "the power of vitamins". Was that a lot of media hype?

Thanks FI. For decades, there has been a gathering of evidence that vitamins, minerals, and other nutrients in our diets have a dramatic impact on our health. Furthermore, some studies show that concentrated forms of these nutrients can be used to prevent and even treat some conditions. Finally a conference of world class scientists was hosted by the New York Academy of Sciences. Essentially, they said that folacin can nearly eliminate a common birth defect, neural tube defect; that vitamin K can probably halt the loss of bone stores, that vitamin E is crucial for preventing heart disease, and other nutrients deserve more attention in modern health care. Used properly, nutrition affords us a very safe, practical, inexpensive, and effective tool to deal with a wide variety of ailments.

Chapter 3

📖

HEALTH TIPS

☞ "My people are destroyed from lack of knowledge." Hosea 4:6

"This is Dr. Patrick Quillin. Join me for health tips each weekday here on the Oasis network. For the next few weeks, my wife Noreen will share secrets on creating meals that are nutritious and delicious. Health tips is heard Monday through Friday at 8:15 am and 4:15 pm."

(opening) This is Health Tips & I'm Dr. Patrick Quillin.
*And I'm Noreen Quillin
Todays question comes from___.   Thanks ___.
(closing) God Bless and good health.

-more fiber in the diet
GR of Broken Arrow. I keep hearing more about fiber and regularity these days, which my grandma talked about a half a century ago. Where can we get fiber?

Fiber is basically found in plant food, not in animal food. Bran and other cereals containing 2-5 grams per serving are a good start on the day. Fruit, vegetables, beans, sea vegetables, and even nuts are all rich sources of fiber. Good health seems to start with regular elimination, meaning at least one soft stool per day. You can use whole grain flour in your cookies, cakes, gravies, and breads for added fiber. A low fiber intake has 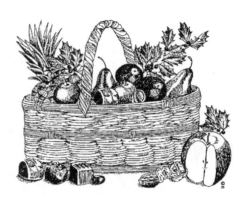 been linked to most of the diseases that Americans suffer from. Your grandma is right. Fiber is nature's broom that keeps our insides healthy and clean.

-cutting the fat in cooking
NT of Midwest City. My diet seems to consist of lots of fried foods, which I know are bad for me. Any suggestions on healthy substitutions?

Most experts agree that too much fat or the wrong kind of fat is a culprit in many diseases, including overweight, heart disease, cancer, and even arthritis. Try substituting plain muffins for doughnuts, unbuttered popcorn for peanuts, baked or barbecued chicken instead of fried, low cal mayonnaise for regular mayo, homemade oil and vinegar dressing for blue cheese, low fat frozen yogurt for ice cream, lean flank steak for rib roast or prime rib, lean pork tenderloin for spareribs, skim milk for whole milk, angel food cake for chocolate cake. Favor olive and canola oil and use less of it. Favor tub margarine or butter over stick margarine. Your efforts at the table will bear fruit in better health and more energy.

-juicing and more plant food

WT of Owasso. Everybody seems to be juicing these days. Is it worth the effort? Anything I need to know before starting?

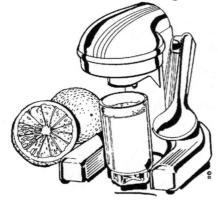

Scientists have recognized more and more special nutrients in plant food that protect us from a variety of diseases. Juicing is a way of consuming more of these valuable nutrients, like beta-carotene, indoles, and chlorophyll. Juicing is okay if you do it in addition to, not instead of, eating good whole fruits and vegetables. If you cannot buy organic produce, then you will need to wash or peel the produce before juicing. The fresher the juice the better. Carrot and apple juice mixed equally is a great juice. 2 or 3 glasses daily taken with meals is a good guideline. You don't need an expensive juicer.

-artificial sweeteners

TC of Oklahoma City. I'm trying to cut down on my sugar intake, but hear unhealthy reports about artificial sweeteners. Any advice?

You are right about the unhealthy track record of artificial sweeteners, although small amounts for most people are probably okay. Better to gradually wean your taste buds of the loads of sweet things that Americans eat. In some people, NutraSweet has created everything from mild headaches to seizures if taken in large quantities, according to studies at MIT. Saccharin is not much better, as it raises the risk for cancer. Sorbitol and mannitol do have calories but do not cause cavities, hence are a limited advantage. We have become a nation of hummingbirds, constantly sipping sweet things that are harmful to our health. Taste the real food instead.

-substitutes for sugar

WK of Sapulpa. What can I substitute for sugar?

If the word "sugar" is on the label, then the product must, by law, be at least 96% processed, with all useful nutrients removed. Other foods that are sweet, but have some redeeming value include: honey, barley malt, concentrated apple juice, fructose, molasses, maltose, fruit juice, date sugar, rice syrup, dates, and apple butter. A product called Succanat is sugar cane that has not been refined, and hence cannot be called sugar, but is quite sweet. Molasses is a decent source of chromium, which improves blood glucose regulation.   Cut the sugar called for in the recipe in half, then work downward from there.   If a spoonful of sugar helps the medicine or healthy food go down, then so be it.   But don't overdo a sweet thing.

-how to change junk food eating habits
OK of Tulsa.   I come from a long line of junk food enthusiasts, and my family's health seems to suffer accordingly.   What can I do to change my eating habits?

Start off by using 2/3 the sugar called for in recipes.   Use half whole grain flour rather than all white flour.   Use brown rice instead of white rice. Use more herbs and spices rather than covering your food with the harmful flavorings of sugar, salt, and fat.   Bake and microwave foods rather than frying.   Get a healthy cookbook, such as the American Cancer Society cookbook.   Learn to read labels when you grocery shop.   When you eat at restaurants, fill up on the salad bar of fresh fruits and vegetables before you get to the entree.   Chose foods from the menu that are baked and broiled, rather than fried and sauteed.   Make gradual changes.   Reward yourself for your progress, no matter how small.   Keep up the good work.

-whole grain versus white flour
WK of Shawnee.   Is enriched white flour good for you?

Compared to whole unprocessed wheat flour, white flour is a mere skeleton of the original nutrients.   The most commonly eaten food in

America is white flour in bread and crackers. To make white flour, the miller must remove the outer bran and inner germ and the 24 nutrients that go with these parts. Then, 4 nutrients are added back to give white flour the misleading name of "enriched". Only 16% of Americans enjoy the wholesome goodness and nutrition that comes with whole grain wheat flour. For a real taste treat, try some whole grain bread from rye, barley, oats, rice, or millet. For each cup of white flour called for in the recipe, substitute one cup of whole grain flour minus one tablespoon, to allow for the water absorbing properties of the bran. Follow the main rule of nutrition, "eat foods in as close to their natural state as possible".

-best cooking methods
JA of Ponca City. Since my dad's heart attack, I am making a serious effort to serve him nutritious foods. What cooking methods lose the most nutrients?

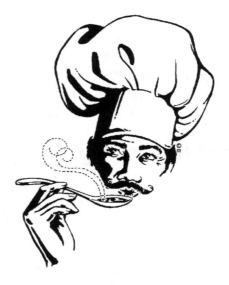

Food begins to degrade the moment it is harvested, so fresh is best. The higher the fluid content, the quicker the deterioration, such as fruits and vegetables. Nutrients are lost through exposure to heat, light, air, moisture, and even iron utensils. Dried plant food, such as beans, nuts, and seeds are designed by God to last until they can bring forth a new crop, so these are more hardy. Cooking in water, then discarding the water is probably the worst method of cookery for nutrient loss. Microwaving, steaming, pressure cooking, roasting, and broiling are the best.

-healthy snacks

LJ of Jenks. I am trying to come up with some healthy TV snacks for my family. Your help please.

You can buy an inexpensive microwave popcorn popper and make cheap, tasty, low fat, high fiber popcorn--without the butter, of course. You can mix whole grain cereals, such as Wheat Chex, Shreaded wheat, and Cheerios, with all bran and sprinkle in some peanuts. You can cut up whole wheat tortillas into strips, then bake in the oven for 8 minutes to make your own healthy chips. You can make a chip dip out of yogurt with dry onion soup mix. You can present them with a bowl of fresh fruit or frozen yogurt. Congratulations on your efforts to make TV time a bit healthier.

-after school snacks for kids

TM of Wagoner. My kids come home hungry from school. Should I give them snacks, or make them wait until dinner?

If your family eats late, then the children may be too hungry to wait. You may consider feeding the kids an early dinner, then let them have dessert with the family later. Or, there are healthy snacks you could provide, such as carrots dipped in peanut butter, or frozen orange sections, or frozen yogurt popsickles, or a trail mix of Shredded Wheat with nuts and raisins. You might even try making your own cookies with whole wheat flour, oats, and peanut butter. Snacking on sugary junk food just before meals often ruins the kids appetites and makes meal time less enjoyable.

-bulk cooking to help when home hungry from work
TK of Sand Springs. I come home from work late, hungry, and tired and usually don't feel like cooking for my family. Any suggestions?

Pick a few hours a week to prepare food in bulk, including pressure cooked whole brown rice, beans, barley, cole slaw, healthy cookies, etc. Cook in bulk and store food in serving size amounts in baggies in freezer. Buy turkey and ham and keep slices in freezer. Turkey hot dogs on whole wheat buns micowaved are a quick and decent meal. Baked chicken and potato require no more than placing in the oven for 40 minutes. Make bulk cookie dough and freeze in cookie size amounts. Keep a large bowl of salad fixings in the refrigerator, such as carrot and cabbage cole slaw, or tossed green salad.

-are eggs healthy?

MT of Miami. Are eggs okay to eat?

For many years, the cholesterol in eggs was

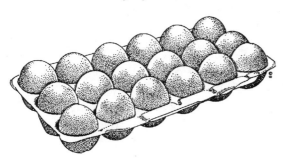

thought to be the villain in America's epidemic of heart disease. But after 20 years of research, the truth shows that total fat, and more importantly oxidized fat in the bloodstream is much more critical than dietary cholesterol. Less than 10% of the population needs to worry about the cholesterol in eggs. According to 15 years of heart disease research on thousands of people, adequate vitamin E intake is much more important than avoiding eggs. Exercise, no smoking, and stress are all important factors in the formula of who gets heart disease. Eggs are cheap, nutritious, easy to cook, and easy to chew.

-coffee, breast lumps, and coffee substitutes

AM of Bartlesville. My doctor has warned me that the non-cancerous lumps in my breast may be caused by too much coffee. What can I drink instead of my precious coffee?

You are not alone in your coffee addiction. Some people actually experience headaches when withdrawing from coffee. Try coffee substitutes found in grocery and health food stores, including

Cafix, Postum, chicory, herbal teas, and Japanese green tea (which actually may help to prevent cancer). While 2 cups of coffee per day for normal healthy adults is probably okay, millions of sensitive individuals develop wild swings in blood sugar and energy levels, or even fibrocystic breast disease. Some people who crave the pick-me-up from coffee may be suffering from low thyroid. Have your doctor examine you. Once you get used to it, green tea with honey and powdered vitamin C is both tasty, refreshing, and quite healthy.

-dessert ideas
LY of Bixby. I need some special dessert recipe that will taste good but be nutritious also.

Try blending chocolate low fat frozen yogurt, then pouring it into a whole wheat pie crust and freeze it. The resulting chocolate pie will make most people want more, and it has some nutritional redeeming qualities. You can also take a fruit pie recipe, substitute whole wheat for the crust, add fresh apples or other fruit and likely please everyone. Another favorite is whole wheat cake bottom with some cocoa added, then make the frosting from yogurt with powdered milk and powder sugar for thickening. Another blue ribbon desert is yogurt with chocolate pudding mix added, then pour this mixture into whole grain pita bread for a chocolate moose taste.

-quick breakfast ideas

GD of Okmulgee. My family just doesn't have time for breakfast, even though we know it would be good for us. Any suggestions?

There are a number of instant powder protein drinks that would suffice for a quick breakfast. Just add these mixes to water, milk, or fruit juice in the blender and you have the quickest take-it-with-you breakfast possible. Also, a number of ready to eat cereals are quite nourishing. Pour milk over Shredded Wheat, Wheat Chex, Cheerios, or any other predominantly whole grain cereal and you have a quick and effective solution to your problem. There are even nutritious granola bars that you can eat on the run. A half century of research shows that people who eat a decent breakfast are far better achievers both at school and the office. Don't leave home without breakfast.

Chapter 4

📖

HEALTH TIPS

☞ "You know you are getting older when all the names in your little black book end with 'M.D.'" Robert Orben, comedian

(opening) "This is health tips and I'm Dr. Patrick Quillin. Today's question comes from..."
(closing) "God bless and good health"

-valerian & sleep
    KB of Okmulgee. I travel a lot and have a hard time sleeping in hotels. I don't like the groggy feeling from sleeping pills but need something to help me sleep. Any suggestions?
    While exercise, a light evening meal, and a peaceful prayer session can help bring on sleep, I sympathize with your problem

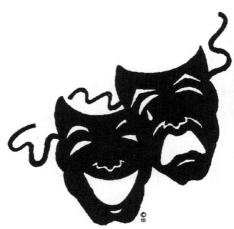

since I also travel a great deal. Good clinical studies have found that a natural herb, valerian, can provide restful sleep without that hangover feeling that comes from sleeping pills. 2-3 capsules of valerian taken one half hour before bedtime on an empty stomach will likely solve your sleeping problem.

-confusion of what is a good diet
RH of Sand Springs. There are more experts on nutrition than fleas on a dog. One person says we should be vegetarians, another says macrobiotic, another says we should only eat raw food, another talks about the four food groups. Can you make some sense out of this nonsense?

Your confusion is understandable RH. Just as most creatures on earth have their own specific diet, humans were created with a Divine design or what scientists call the Paleolithic diet. Our early ancestors ate a bland diet consisting of lean meat from active animals and the remaining calories from unprocessed plants, like vegetables, nuts, grains, beans, and fruit. If you follow this Divine design of eating a wide variety of meals that are one third low fat meat and two thirds fresh plant food, then you will cut through all the controversy in nutrition.

-healthy fats for dog's coat and human skin
KT of South Tulsa. My grandpa has two hunting dogs with beautiful fur and good health. He says that their special dog food along with some

fresh avocados help their coat. Does nutrition also help people's skin?

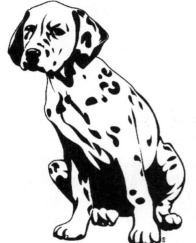

Very perceptive KT. "You are what you eat" is a very accurate statement. The only other creatures on earth with the same health problems as Americans are our domestic pets, since the pets sometimes are treated to the same junk food. The skin, hair, and nails on any animal are a direct reflection of that creature's general health. Veterinarians are keenly aware of the importance of diet in the health of animals. The skin is considered a sacrificial organ in most animals and thus is the first tissue to suffer with any form of malnutrition or stress. The right amount of protein, fatty acids (such as from fish), zinc, vitamin C, and other nutrients will help to insure healthy coats in animals and attractive clear complexions in humans. If you knew how particular the diet is for rare zoo pets and expensive race horses, then we all might be a little more attentive to the nutrition needs of our bodies.

-healthier seasonings

TT of Claremore. My husband recently had a heart attack and the doctor says no more sugar, salt, or fat to cook with. What am I supposed to season the food with to make him eat. He is beside himself with depression.

Americans have developed a very dangerous habit of using sugar, fat, and salt to season foods. Just as we developed this habit, we can also change it. Change takes a 3 week commitment to the adjustment period. Instead of deep frying meats, try broiling, baking, or grilling. Steam or microwave your vegetables. Use ginger, garlic, onions, soy sauce, mustard, peppers, parsley, sage, thyme, mint, cloves, and olive oil for seasonings. Get the American Cancer Society cookbook to get started on this new healthy lifestyle. Be patient and you will soon revel in the new found flavors in your food.

-heart disease & blood cholesterol

TM of Bartlesville. My grandpa has been ordered to lower his cholesterol or probably face another heart attack. We have cut out eggs from the diet and he is on medication, but still having problems getting his cholesterol down. Your help please.

There are many nutrients that affect the serum cholesterol level, including favorable influences from: vitamin E, chromium picolinate, carnitine, vitamin C, niacin, fish oil, ginger, chicory, and fiber; with negative impact from stress, sedentary lifestyle, tobacco, and high fat diet. Dietary cholesterol has minimal impact on serum cholesterol, so eggs are okay for most people. The real improvements in serum cholesterol come from lowering total fat intake, exercise, relaxation, and supplements of the nutrients mentioned.

-can't afford book, want information for free

CP of Jenks. I can't afford to buy any of your books. Where can I get some good nutrition information for free?

My books are also available in the Tulsa library system, as are many other good nutrition books; including: Nutritional Influences on Illness by Dr. Mel Werbach, The Doctor's Vitamin and Mineral Encyclopedia by Dr. Sheldon Hendler, Encyclopedia of Natural Medicine by Dr. Mike Murray, and more. You may also call Bronson Pharmaceuticals at 1-800-235-3200 and request a free copy of my Nutrition Encyclopedia, which is a handy reference guide. Money should not be an obstacle to good health. Actually, the average family of 4 will save $1500 annually in food bills by eating a healthier diet.

-larger breakfast, smaller dinner

OR of Bixby. I remember my Grandma telling us to "eat breakfast like a king, lunch like a prince, and dinner like a pauper" Is there any truth to this?

Yes. Good studies show that a large meal or a high fat meal consumed late in the day before bedtime is more likely to cause heart disease and much more likely to become body fat. Eat your last meal of the day at least 2 hours before bedtime and make it a reasonably small meal. Much of the fat that we eat at dinner will end up being deposited in our arteries for future heart disease or in the fatty tissue for immediate weight problems. Your Grandma was right.

-fluid intake with meal

BR of Oklahoma City. My kids drink a gallon of iced kool aid nearly every supper. Is that alright?

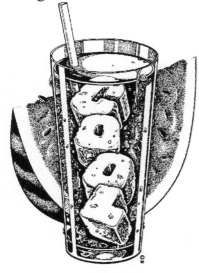

Actually, no. while we all need large amounts of clean fluids daily, when we drink too much fluids at mealtime, we make it hard for the body to digest and absorb the nutrients from the food. Realize that your body must manufacture an impressive collection of strong acid and enzymes to breakdown the food into nutrients that are absorbed. Drinking large amounts of fluid at mealtime dilutes these critical acids and enzymes and lowers the efficiency of the intestines. Better to have most of your fluids a half hour before or one hour after mealtime. As far as temperature of mealtime beverages, best to drink warm fluids like herb tea, coffee substitutes, hot chocolate or hot apple cider, to help disperse fats and fat soluble vitamins for better absorption.

-athletes & need for fluids and electrolytes

JT of Midwest City. My daughter is a high school basketball player. She often complains of muscle cramps during and after her practice sessions. Any suggestions?

Yes. Muscle cramps are often caused by dehydration, or electrolyte depletion, or vitamin E deficiency. Make sure that you are eating foods high in potassium (from cantaloupe, apricots, bananas, broccoli, fruits, and vegetables), also magnesium (from wheat germ, whole grains, molasses, soybeans, shrimp, spinach, and peas), calcium (from yogurt, collards, turnip greens, kale), and vitamin E (from wheat germ and whole grains). For athletes who lose a lot of electrolytes and fluid in sweat, you may need to provide supplements, like the potassium/magnesium liquid product sold in health food stores.

-young athletes, weight loss & growth stunting

MP of Porter. My son is in high school wrestling and these boys are always starving themselves. Is that good for a growing boy?

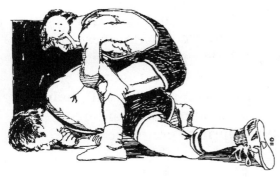

No. Studies show that by depriving a growing adolescent of just 1% of their calorie needs that growth stunting will result. While organized athletics and exercise are wonderful for teens, starving a growing person to "make weight" in wrestling is very unhealthy. Growth stunting means that the body and brain will not reach their genetic potential for size and health. Pick a reasonable weight for your boy to wrestle at and raise that weight as he shows signs of growing. While the usual teenage "eat-everything in the refrigerator" syndrome is unnecessary, growing teenagers need proper nutrition to produce a healthy adult.

-vegetarian diet & need for complimentary proteins

BK of Wagoner. My daughter is pregnant with her first baby and insists that her vegetarian eating habits won't hurt the baby. What do you think?

A vegetarian diet can be healthy, if you do it right. Vegetarians are prone toward deficiencies in protein, iron, zinc, B-6, and carnitine. Healthy vegetarianism means getting complementary proteins from a mixture of grains and beans (like whole wheat tortillas with beans or a peanut butter sandwich). While it is possible to deliver a healthy baby from a vegetarian mother, it takes some forethought and effort. The richest sources of protein in plant food include: garbanzo beans, soybeans in tempeh and tofu, wheat germ, brewer's yeast, and spirulina. Adequate protein will help to prevent the bloating and toxemia that often set in with protein deficiency during pregnancy.

-water purifier & bottled water
TM of Muskogee. With all the newspaper articles I read about toxic spills, I'm getting a little concerned about our drinking water in Oklahoma. Do I need a water filterer for my family home?

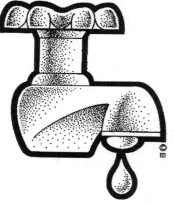

Probably. the Environmental Protection Agency has called our water pollution issue" a ticking time bomb" and "a national disgrace". Unfortunately, we have spent the last century dumping some very potent poisons into our rivers, lakes, and underground aquifers. While we all should make efforts to recycle and elect environmentally responsible politicians, we should also drink purified water. You can buy a reverse osmosis system for $300 that will remove nearly all pollutants from your drinking water. Or you can buy bottled water from a reputable dealer. Boiling water will kill bacteria but not remove toxins. Since two thirds of your body weight is water, a lifetime of consuming polluted water can have a harmful impact on your health.

-cancer scare & prevention

RR of Miami. In the last year I lost six friends and family members to cancer. Is there something I can do to protect myself against this disease?

Most definitely. Experts tell us that from 50% to 90% of all cancer is induced by lifestyle and preventable. Don't smoke. Avoid obesity. If you drink, do so in moderation. Drink purified water not tap water. Watch for pollutants in both the home and workplace. Keep a happy outlook on life. Eat less sugar and fat while consuming more fresh fruits and vegetables. Take a broad spectrum vitamin and mineral supplement with adequate levels of selenium, beta-carotene, vitamin E, and C. Eat enough fiber to insure daily bowel movements that float. Have regular medical exams or at least do self breast and testicle exams. If you have a strange lump or bump, get it checked by your doctor. Better that you don't get cancer at all, but cancer that is detected early has a much better chance of being cured.

-ginger & motion sickness

BT of Sapulpa. My kids seem to get sick on car and boat rides. Any nutrition things I can do to help them with motion sickness?

Yes. In double blind studies, pills of the herb ginger have been proven to reduce motion sickness as effectively as prescription drugs. Ginger is a wonder herb that also helps to prevent heart disease and cancer. Buy fresh ginger root in the produce section of your grocery store, freeze it, then pull it out and grate it for a spicey flavoring in many foods. For your kids motion sickness, take 2 ginger capsules 30 minutes before getting in the car or boat. Through plants, God has provided us with many effective and non-toxic approaches to make our life better.

-simple guidelines for healthy eating
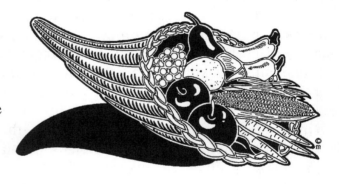
    DW of Oolagah. I've been listening to your Health Tips for almost 2 years now and I appreciate what you have done for my family's health. Are there some real simple rules to help my husband eat better?

    Most definitely. Eat foods in as close to their natural state as possible. God's food is always better than mankinds refined version of that food. Eat a wide variety of foods, not focusing on any particular food. Eat small frequent meals. Eat enough calories to maintain a decent weight. Shop the perimeter of the grocery store. If your food will not rot or sprout, then don't eat it; because if a bacteria is not interested in that food, then what makes you think that your body cells are going to be nourished by it. Eat to live, don't live to eat.

-Scriptural basis

AR of Grove. You have a lot of good ideas about nutrition, but do they have any Scriptural basis? What does the Bible say about nutrition?

Plenty. In Genesis 1:29. we find: Behold I have given you every plant & it shall be food for you. Genesis 1:12. And the earth brought forth vegetation and God saw that it was good". Indeed, a diet that is based on high vegetable intake will lower the risk for about every major disease faced by Americans. Also, one third of all prescription drugs are derived from plant extracts and more uses are being found each day for the wonderful pharmacy found in the plant kingdom. Jesus fed the multitudes fish and whole grain bread, not pizza and soft drinks. 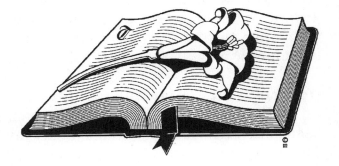 Fasting is mentioned throughout the Bible. Indeed modern scientists find that the one nutrition habit that will best insure good health and long life is undernutrition without malnutrition. Nourishing Ezekial bread is made from a recipe in the Old Testament. Since a sick body inhibits a life of worship and service, the Bible is telling us to feed both your spirit and body what they need.

-irregular heartbeat & magnesium

WT of Oklahoma City. My husband has been having problems with irregular heart beat. His doctor wants to put in a pacemaker, but my husband is so young for that. What should we do?

You should work with your doctor. And there are some less drastic possibilities that may clear up the problem without the need for surgery. Eating foods and supplements that are high in potassium (2 grams/day), plus magnesium (600 mg), plus calcium (600 mg), plus coenzyme Q (100 mg), plus a broad spectrum vitamin supplement while cutting back on salt intake may help revitalize the heart back into regular pumping rhythm. Physicians find that 90% of all heart attack victims have abnormally low levels of serum magnesium. Work with your doctor and see if these simple non-toxic techniques may help before plunging into surgery.

-feverfew & migraine headaches

FT of Ponca City. I get these migraine headaches that just about make my eyes pop out. The drugs that help also leave me feeling like a zombie. Any options?

Yes. Feverfew is an herb that was once thought to reduce fever, which it probably doesn't. However, in a double blind study reported in the British Medical Journal, 3 capsules of feverfew were able to help two thirds of migraine sufferers. Also, magnesium supplements of 600 mg/day have been independently shown to prevent or reduce migraines.

-chromium & extended lifespan

PK of Shawnee. My grandma lived to a ripe age of 96 and claimed that her frequent walks and daily cube of brewer's yeast were her longevity secrets. Any truth to granny's theory?

Yes. Ten years worth of research from Tufts University in Boston has shown that aging can be seriously delayed with fitness. The most important indicator of your biological age is percent body fat. Pinch the skin just above your hip bone. If you have more than an inch, then you need to embark on an exercise program. Granny's walks were shear magic for lowering blood lipids, improving heart function, and lowering percent body fat--which essentially keeps you younger longer. Brewer's yeast is one of the richest sources of chromium, which is critical for the proper burning of blood glucose. Without adequate chromium, we develop diabetes-like symptoms and heart disease. In a recent study, animals that were given chromium supplements lived 1/3 longer than their non-supplemented peers, which would equate to a 20 or 30 year life extension in humans. We all could profit from granny's walk and brewer's yeast.

-memory & ginkgo

OW of Broken Arrow. I am only 45 and my memory seems to be fading badly. I need help.

Point well taken. The brain is vulnerable to both poor nutrition, poor health, and exposure to toxins. The brain needs regular mental stimulation, plus a constant flow of oxygen rich blood to function well. Unfortunately, many Americans, even at your age, are well en route toward blocked vessels and the brain is literally starving to death. Check with your doctor. While you work on a diet and lifestyle that will unplug your blood vessels, there is an herb ginkgo biloba that has been clinically proven to improve blood flow to the brain and other peripheral tissue. 120 mg daily of ginkgo improves memory for many people.

Chapter 5

📖

HEALTH TIPS

☞ "We live in a world of problems which can no longer be solved by the level of thinking which created them." Albert Einstein

(opening) "This is health tips and I'm Dr. Patrick Quillin. Today's question comes from..."
(closing) "God bless and good health."

-beans and "wind"
NT of Broken Arrow. You have mentioned the health value of beans, but frankly I have a lot of gas when I eat beans. Any suggestions?
An uncomfortable but very common problem. Gas from beans is a result of bacteria in the intestines fermenting the beans rather than your digestive tract being able to digest and absorb the beans. You can lessen the problem by first bringing dry uncooked beans to a boil for 2 minutes, then turn off burner and let stand on the stove for an hour while covered. Drain off the water, then cook in pressure cooker for 20-30 minutes. Also, use yogurt, garlic, ginger, and mustard at the same meal

to reduce gas. The more often that you eat beans, the more your body produces the enzymes necessary to process the beans. For a temporary help, use the patented product "Beano" which provides the missing enzyme that make beans more tolerable to you and your company.

-calcium & osteoporosis

GR of Midwest City. My mother suffered badly from osteoporosis and I want to avoid it. How much calcium should I take?

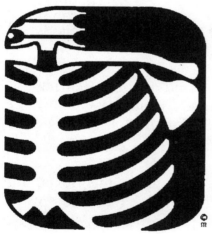

Calcium is the most publicized part of the problem, but just a piece of the puzzle in osteoporosis. Many risk factors contribute to osteoporosis, or hollowing of the bones: sedentary lifestyle, since the force of gravity encourages solid bones; psychological stress as in the Biblical passage "a merry heart does good, but a broken spirit dries up the bones"; alcohol; tobacco; excess protein or phosphorus in the diet will increase risks while, too little calcium, vitamin D, or magnesium are also well known risk factors. Your best lifestyle to avoid osteoporosis would include exercise, a well balanced diet, positive attitude, and supplements of multiple vitamins, bone meal, epsom salts, and cod liver oil.

-arthritis & allergies

TC of Owasso. My wife suffers terribly from arthritis and the doctors can't seem to help much. Any advice?

While arthritis is rarely fatal, it is often crippling. 20 million Americans suffer from some form of arthritis. One study found that 75% of arthritis sufferers experienced dramatic relief when they ate a diet free of common allergenic foods. Allergies can cause many seemingly unrelated symptoms, including arthritis, headaches, diabetes, behavioral disorders, and even heart disease. Other nutritional approaches to arthritis include supplements of fish oil and anti-oxidants, which help to reduce inflammation. Other studies have shown benefit from pantothenic acid or royal bee jelly, ginger, vitamin C, niacinamide, zinc, copper, and even topically applied DMSO.

-water pollution & purifier

WT of Oklahoma City. I'm becoming more concerned about water pollution in this country. How can I protect my family.

Even the conservative governmental group, the Environmental Protection Agency, is concerned about water pollution, calling the situation: "a ticking time bomb". While we all can make efforts to clean up our own back yard and elect environmentally responsible politicians, we also need to protect ourselves from the likelihood of contaminated drinking water which can increase the risk for cancer, heart disease, birth defects, and allergies. It is wise to drink either commercially filtered water purchased in the store, or filter your own water at home. I prefer home filtered water for convenience and cost, with the best system being reverse osmosis, followed by solid block carbon filtration unit, then distillation. With respect to water pollution, ignorance of the facts may jeopardize you and your family.

-alcohol during pregnancy

OM of Sapulpa. My son and daughter have several glasses of wine every night and she is pregnant. I tell them that alcohol doesn't mix with pregnancy and they tell me how everyone in the Bible drank wine. Your insight please.

One of the most common birth defects in Western society is fetal alcohol syndrome, which is totally caused by alcohol intake during pregnancy, is entirely preventable, and is a permanent defect on the child. While many people in the Bible drank wine, none of them were pregnant. Scientists recommend abstaining from alcohol intake during pregnancy because they don't know what level of 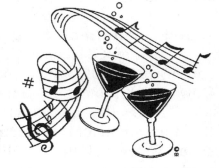 alcohol intake might be considered safe. Fetal alcohol syndrome can be blatant, such as children who look somewhat like Down's sydrome kids, or it can be much more subtle, like minor defects in behavior, mental abilities, or urinary tract problems. Best advice: don't drink alcohol when pregnant.

-heart palpitations & nutrients

KW of Miami. At age 40, I've been starting back into an exercise program, but have had some heart palpitations. My doctor can't find anything wrong with my heart, but this continues to happen when I exercise. Your help please.

The heart is an amazing muscle that serves us without rest for many decades. You can help this vital organ with some nutrition tips. Muscles contract with the help of calcium, and relax with magnesium and potassium. Many Americans lack adequate calcium, magnesium, and potassium in the diet. You can increase your intake of whole grains, soybeans, and dark green vegetables. You might also consider a nutrition supplement called Liquid K Plus, which contains potassium and magnesium in very bioavailable forms. Add some calcium from egg shell or bone meal and you have minerals that should help prevent heart palpitations.

-sore back & legs from too much standing

WM of Tulsa. I work all day standing on my feet and by the time I get home, my legs, feet, and back are killing me. Any advice.

You are likely suffering from poor circulation and stress on delicate joints. Blood can collect in the feet and lower legs if there is no muscle movement to help return the blood to the heart, which is fighting gravity. While you are working during the day, do toe raises regularly to keep the lower leg muscles moving the blood back to the heart. Wear comfortable shoes and support hose. When you get home try two things, first place a chinup bar securely in the house or garage so that you can hang from this bar. Let your back muscles and joints relax and stretch out. Next, lie on the floor with your lower legs up on the padded ottoman. Press your lower back to the floor several times, then rest.

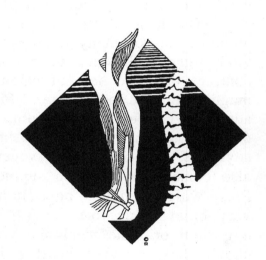

-vitamin E preventing sore muscles
JA of Shawnee. After a twenty year break in my exercise program, I recently returned to daily running, but find morning stiffness is a serious problem. Any suggestions.

While exercise can be very good for you, it is also very stressful on the body. Researchers find that people who provide their body with the necessary nutrients will reap more benefits and less damage from exercise. For instance, studies show that vitamin E supplements of about 400 iu/day will reduce exercise induced damage and the stiffness that comes with pushing muscles beyond their limit. Anti-oxidants, like vitamin E, C, and beta-carotene can protect against the higher exposure to oxygen that comes with exercise. Also, note the increased need for magnesium, calcium, potassium, zinc, and chromium that comes with regular workouts. With a little nutritional forethought you can make exercise a major positive force in your life.

-symptoms of low thyroid

BT of Sand Springs. My daughter is having painful periods, just like I used to have. I am now on thyroid medication. Do you think my daughter could benefit from thyroid?

You need to have your daughter examined by a physician. Yes, low thyroid has a tendency to run in families and can be the culprit in painful menstruation. Low thyroid occurs in about 40% of the population with symptoms including: fertility problems or painful menstrual cycles, easy weight gain, lethargy, sluggish mind, frequent coldness, and constipation. Millions of people struggle through a lack luster life when simple and non toxic thyroid supplements would provide amazing relief. If your morning temperature is less than 97.8 degrees Fahrenheit, then you are a likely candidate for thyroid replacement therapy.

-zinc & appetite in older adults

JM of Jenks. My mother has been living with us for a few years now and she seems to be losing her appetite. I am concerned that she may be suffering from malnutrition. What should we do?

As we mature, we oftentimes develop a loss of taste buds, or hypogusia, which can be the beginning of a series of events that lead to illness. Older adults are particularly at risk for the loss of taste sensation. Taking 30-50 mg/day of zinc picolinate for 1 month will sometimes restore these lost taste buds to near normal. It is always best to take vitamin and mineral supplements in a comprehensive package with a reasonable balance of all the right nutrients. Lost taste buds can begin poor eating habits, which can begin health troubles from clinical malnutrition. For instance, older adults are more likely to load their food with sugar and salt, since their taste buds are less sensitive. Studies have found that 90% of institutionalized older adults were suffering from scurvy, or severe vitamin C deficiency. Proper nutrition is important at all stages of life, including older adulthood.

-diabetes and diet

CW of Norman. I developed adult diabetes somewhat around my 50th birthday and have not had to use insulin yet. Will I remain on this oral medication forever?

In a fascinating study published in the journal Diabetes in 1986, a group of Australian researchers gathered 10 adult diabetic volunteers who were

Aboriginals living in the city. The researchers asked these Aborigines to return to the native hunting and gathering lifestyle of their ancestors. Within 7 weeks, all patients had dramatically improved health, with lowered serum cholesterol, an average of 18 pounds lost in spite of no efforts at weight loss, and essentially all were cured of their diabetes. In many adult diabetics, a little effort at weight loss, dietary control, and minimal exercise can bring about tremendous improvements in general health.

-help for low sperm count

LQ of Okmulgee. My husband and I are eager to start a family, but have had problems. Our doctor says that my husband's sperm count might be too low to have children. Any help?

Just like everything else in the body, sperm is built from the nutrients in your diet. Studies have shown dramatic improvement in both quantity and quality of sperm when subjects consumed more vitamin C. Supplements of 1000 mg/day cut sperm clumping by 2/3 in 35 infertile men. In a separate study, 39% of the 178 infertile men studied experienced improvements in sperm count with 10 grams/day of the amino acid arginine. Also, beware that the gonads function best when operating somewhat below body temperature, hence hot tubs and tight cotton pants and underwear can lower fertility.

-colic in baby & milk allergy in mother

NV of Bartlesville. My new baby is having a terrible time with colic. I am breastfeeding, so don't think that she is getting air bubbles. Any suggestions?

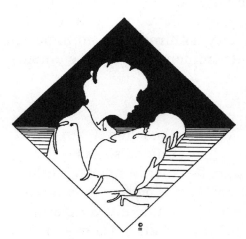

Small amounts of your food intake will pass into your infant's breast milk and could account for the problem. For instance, remove strong tasting foods, like garlic, onions, broccoli, and brussel sprouts. Caffeine should be entirely removed, which means coffee, tea, colas, chocolate, and certain medications. Also, mother and infant seem to exchange the makings of an allergy. In a published study, one third of colicky babies got better when their nursing mothers stopped consuming dairy products. Since cow's milk is the most common allergenic food, it makes sense that mother's allergy to milk would irritate her nursing infant.

-help in quitting smoking

CA of Wagoner. I have been smoking for 22 years and have the worst time trying to quit. My body just doesn't want to exist without tobacco. Any help.

There are a number of medical programs, like nicotine patches, that can help. Also, hypnosis has 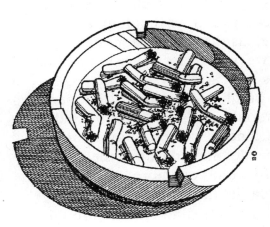 helped thousands of smokers to quit. But for some smokers, its almost like tobacco is an essential vitamin that their body can't live without. For these people, low basal metabolism may be the problem. Tobacco elevates basal metabolism, elevating pulse and the rate at which the smoker burns calories. This brings about a heightened sense of well being and energy, which leaves when tobacco is discontinued. Yet, you can replace the hazards of tobacco with the benefits of sea kelp, chromium, and carnitine to elevate basal metabolism in a healthy way.

-malnutrition in America

FW of Claremore. I have enjoyed your Health Tips for years now, but I can't understand how the richest nation on earth with the most productive farmers in history could possibly have any malnourished people.

Hard to believe, but true. The problem is not quantity of food. As you point out, American farmers are the most productive in the history of the world. Yet our food choices are not in keeping with our bodies' needs. Americans chose food for taste, cost, convenience, and a psychological reward. Those reasons are fine, as long as we remember that the main reason we eat is to nourish the body with the raw materials to carry on the life processes. You can't build and continue to operate a factory with junk materials and the wrong kind of fuel. Extensive government surveys have found that 90% of Americans do not consume the recommended intake for one or more nutrients. Malnutrition in America is through poor choices, while other countries have malnutrition through lack of food supplies.

Chapter 6

📖

HEALTH TIPS

☞ "More people have been killed with a fork and spoon than all other weapons combined." Philip Smith, MD

(opening) This is health tips and I'm Dr. Patrick Quillin. Today's question comes from___
(closing) God Bless and good health.

-baby food from blender

MA of Okmulgee. My baby is beginning to eat baby food, but that stuff is so expensive. We want to feed our baby right but we have a tight budget. Any suggestions?

Thanks MA.
Sounds like your baby has very caring parents. Instead of using expensive canned baby food that is somewhat refined and overcooked, I recommend that you puree your foods that you eat from the table. Take several chicken

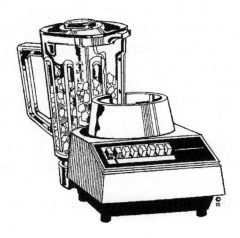

breasts and puree in the blender with some milk, then freeze this liquid food in ice cube trays. Take out one cube at meal time for defrosting. Do the same with fruits, vegetables, whole grains and other foods, only adding milk or liquids if you have to. Make a blender full, then freeze the food in ice cube trays. When baby eats the same good food as the parents, then you not only save considerable money, but you also have much more control over the nutritional quality of your foods.

-how can plant substances help cancer patients?

BK of Broken Arrow. I read in your new book, BEATING CANCER WITH NUTRITION, that America has spent $35 billion in research trying unsuccessfully to find a cure for cancer. Yet you say that simple little old plants can help fight cancer. How?

Thanks BK. While we have all been wowed by the impressive show of antibiotics, laser surgery, and CAT scans; modern medicine is still struggling to find effective therapies against many forms of cancer. Meanwhile, good scientific evidence from the best universities in this country have shown that many plant substances in a wholesome diet will both prevent and help to reverse cancer. Humble little cabbage and broccoli contain a potent phytochemical called indoles, which improve immune functions and help to check the spread of cancer. Garlic, seaweed, carrots, dark green leafy vegetables, citrus fruit, fish and other foods all have their own potent chemicals that fight cancer and other diseases. In Genesis 1:12 we read, "And the earth brought forth vegetation and God saw that it was good." God has developed an assortment of life-giving substances that we are only beginning to appreciate and use. Perhaps the real answer to cancer will lie in good nutrition and prevention.

-flu season at school

HR of Oklahoma City. Its flu season and kids are getting sick all over the place. What can I do to keep my kids from getting the flu?

Good question HR. There are a number of recommendations that will help. Make sure that your kids get plenty of rest and are in good spirits. Stress and fatigue will lower immune response and allow the flu to take hold. Teach your kids to stay away from other kids who are coughing and sneezing. Make sure your kids drink plenty of clean water to flush out the system. Also, nutrients can stimulate the immune system to become even more aggressive against flu bugs. Give your kids a broad spectrum vitamin and mineral supplement with an extra gram of vitamin C each day. Include garlic, fish, ginger, hot peppers, and tumeric in their diet often. If you maintain the immune defenses of your body, then you will have fewer and milder bouts of the flu.

-nasal purge and sinus problems

MC of Tulsa. My husband works as a carpenter and gets a nose full of sawdust all day. He suffers terribly from sinus problems and medication doesn't seem to help. We need your advise.

Thanks MC. Allergy sufferers and people who work in dusty professions, listen up. There is a very simple technique that has been used by country doctors for centuries to help sinus problems. Its called the "nasal purge" and it involves trying to duplicate the conditions of swimming in the ocean. Dissolve 1/2 teaspoon of salt in 1 cup of lukewarm water. Gently and slowly draw the salt water up into your sinus passages by slowly inhaling. Then, plug your nose for a few seconds, then expel whatever comes out. As in swimming, you are trying to force water into the sinuses, but not the lungs. Do this technique weekly for general cleansing or daily for people who get a nose full of dust throughout the day. It really works. Also, there are homeopathic preparations at your health food store that help allergy sufferers.

-prostate problems

TS of Bartlesville. I'm a 62 year old male and have been having problems with painful urination. My doctor says I may need surgery to remove my prostate gland if it gets worse.

Thanks TS. You are suffering from a common problem in males over age 40. The prostate gland is a doughnut shaped organ that can pinch off the uretha that allows us to urinate, kind of like stepping on a garden hose. Hollywood stars Bill Bixby and Don Ameche are among the 35,000 American men who died of prostate cancer last year. An enlarged prostate gland may be the early stages of prostate cancer in many men. To help reduce prostate enlargement, eat less meat, more vegetables, take a broad spectrum vitamin and mineral supplement, along with 50 mg of extra zinc, and the herb saw palmetto extract. The problem should improve in 2 weeks. Keep working with your doctor. Prostate problems can become more than an inconvenience.

-Oprah & exchange system

FG of Claremore. I read in a tabloid about the special diet that Oprah Winfrey used to lose 80 pounds and keep it off. This diet looked surprisingly similar to my diabetic exchange list.

Bravo, FG. You are very perceptive and alert. While there are some very valuable scientific methods to help expedite weight loss, there are no magic bullets that allow someone to eat lots of junk food and still lose weight. Oprah, and millions of other women, have lost plenty of weight in their lives. They just don't keep it off. My advice: "Never say diet". Your program has to become a lifetime of healthy living, not just some temporary phase of self-denial. Most importantly, the amount of fat in your diet will directly affect the amount of fat in your body. Therefore, avoid deep fried foods and minimize butter, ice cream, cheese, salad dressings, nuts, and high fat beef. I do believe that Oprah has finally lost it all for good. With something as simple as the exchange system of meal planning, so can you.

-iron, anemia, heart disease & cancer

KJ of Jenks. My husband has cancer and has been told that he is anemic, so he should eat more iron rich foods, like red meat, and take an iron supplement. But he has been a red meat tyrano saurus rex from the day I met him. How could he be anemic?

Good question KJ. Cancer often includes anemia, as the growing tumor captures the body's iron stores and uses it for growth. Also, chemotherapy often reduces the ability of the body to make new red blood cells. Therefore, many cancer patients become anemic. I would be very cautious about adding significant amounts of iron to his diet. While iron is an essential mineral, it also has been shown that people with higher than normal amounts of iron in the body are at greater risk for heart disease and cancer. For adult men, donating blood several times a year becomes a wonderful way to skim off extra iron stores while helping others at the same time. It takes more than just iron to build more red blood cells. Take a broad spectrum supplement which includes no more than 20 mg of iron, some zinc, copper, B-6, B-12, folacin and a separate liver extract supplement. Build the blood supply slowly. You want to feed your husband, not the cancer.

-folacin & pregnancy

NT of Bixby. My daughter-in-law is pregnant again. Her last baby had neural tubes defects and died shortly after birth. Is there something we can do to avoid that heartbreak from happening again?

Thanks NT. There is plenty she can do. Don't drink alcohol or smoke. Don't use drugs, including all but the most essential prescription drugs. Eat a good diet which includes more vegetables and whole grains and avoids the sugar, fat, salt, and chocolate laddened junk food that is so popular in America. Take a broad spectrum supplement with a healthy dose of vitamins and minerals. Most importantly, take an extra 800 micrograms of folacin, a B vitamin. In about a dozen studies examining nearly 10,000 women, folacin was clearly found to nearly eliminate neural tubes defects in 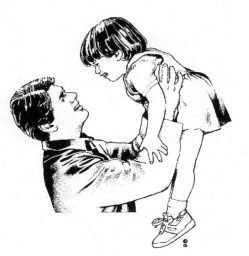 women who were genetically prone toward this problem. The process of creating a baby is quite a miracle. Pregnant women can do their part in making this miracle a successful outcome by feeding their unborn baby a lot of love and good nutrients while avoiding toxins.

-sickness & stress

WP of Midwest City. I always seem to get a cold just before some major holiday comes along. Can you help me?

Yes WP. Holidays can be happy or sad times for people, but they are usually stressful times.

Stress can be both pleasant, like a honeymoon, or unpleasant, like the loss of a loved one. When the mind is stressed, the immune system that protects us from infectigns, becomes less effective. There are nutrients that can bolster the immune system, like zinc, selenium, B-6, and E. There are also emotions that can bolster immune function, like happiness, laughter, creating art or music, expressing yourself in a journal, prayer, meditation, and so on. It sounds to me like the stress, be it good or bad, of having friends and family around at holidays pushes your immune system into a slump. Try some relaxation techniques for the week before holidays. Include a comprehensive health plan of enough sleep, good diet, supplements, and some exercise for stress reduction. Many people get so nervous, or excited, worried, or depressed that they get sick, often at the most inconvenient times of the year, like holidays.

-why should I change eating habits

AL of Sand Springs. My hard headed dad that I love so much won't change his diet, even though his doctor says he is diving straight into a heart attack. He says if his diet hasn't killed him after 50 years of eating this way, then why change now. Maybe you can answer that one.

Thanks AL. Your question cuts right to the heart of the problem. God created humans as very tough and tenacious creatures. Just because we survive something does not mean that it helps us to thrive. No one dies with their first cigarette or alcoholic binge, even though these are very poisonous. It takes decades of exposure to many toxins before they begin to erode your health. It takes decades of low calcium intake before osteoporosis, or hollowing of the bones, will surface; and decades of high fat low fiber diet before heart disease explodes in a stroke or heart attack. Our tough nature becomes our undoing. We spend much of our lives slowly eroding the God-given health that we could be nourishing. Many people eat poorly for decades and assume that since their diet hasn't killed them, then it must be good for them. Too often, it is cancer or a heart attack that finally forces a person to change their unhealthy lifestyle. Don't let your toughness be your downfall.

-breast cancer in family & preventive surgery

LK of Porter. Breast cancer seems to run in my family and my doctor has suggested that I have preventive surgery to remove my healthy breasts, just to avoid the problem. What do you think?

Thanks LK. While preventive breast surgery used to be very popular, it has become less common in recent years, now that we better understand the lifestyle factors which can help a woman avoid breast cancer. Cancer does run in families, hence genetics plays a role. Yet families tend to have similar lifestyles: like eating the same food in the same quantities, or smoking, or living a sedentary lifestyle, or being exposed to the same pollutants from nearby farms or factories. More experts now agree that breast cancer is not the unavoidable consequence of a person's genetics, but more influenced by diet, toxins, and stress. I would strongly suggest that you get my book, BEATING CANCER WITH NUTRITION, or Dr. Simone's book, CANCER AND NUTRITION, to learn the lifestyle factors that will dramatically lower your risk for cancer.

-sugar & cancer

PT of Miami. In your book, BEATING CANCER WITH NUTRITION, you mentioned that sugar can feed cancer. Doesn't bread end up as sugar in the blood? I'm confused.

Good question PT. Cancer appears to be an obligate glucose metabolizer, which means a sugar feeder. High levels of sugar in the blood is like throwing gasoline on a spark to ignite cancer. One way to reduce the risk for cancer or to slow its growth is to limit the amount of fuel available to the tumor. You can do this by regulating blood glucose levels, much the same way that a diabetic does. Never eat anything sweet by itself. If you are going to eat sweet foods, preferably fruits, then eat them with a mixed meal which includes protein, fiber, and fat to modify rises in blood glucose. Seriously limit your intake of refined sugars. Change your taste buds to be less dependent on sweet foods. Take supplements of B-6, zinc, and chromium to improve glucose and insulin metabolism. What you are trying to do is limit the dramatic rises in blood sugar that come with eating sweet foods alone. A high sugar diet is a major risk factor for diabetes, cancer, obesity, heart disease, and other illnesses.

-no time for breakfast

KN of Bixby. I am a busy working mother with 3 kids and simply have no time for breakfast, even though I know we would all be better off if we ate breakfast. Any suggestions?

Yes, KN. After 40 years of research, it is clear that people who eat a nourishing breakfast perform better at school and at work with fewer behavioral problems and mood swings. Ready to eat breakfast cereals made from whole grains and with minimal sugar added are a quick and valuable breakfast, like Shredded Wheat, Cherrios, and Grapenuts. You can even eat these cereals dry, just like a trail mix, while on the way to work. You can mix these cereals with a smaller amount of dry roasted unsalted peanuts for calorie-hungry growing children. The health food store carries a dozen different varieties of health bars that are rich in protein, fiber, vitamins, and minerals and serve as a decent meal replacement. Before you go to bed at night, blend up some powdered protein with carrots and banana and store in the refrigerator for a quick drink next morning. Keep some peeled and boiled eggs in the refrigerator and eat them on the way to work. You are right to be concerned about breakfast.

-need recipes & details on making it work

LC of Owasso. My whole family enjoys your health tips, but we need some recipe ideas on how to make the big change to a healthier diet.

Thanks LC. Yours is the ultimate practical question. In my book, BEATING CANCER WITH NUTRITION, my wife Noreen and I have outlined 2 whole weeks of healthy dining, complete with recipes and meal plans. Valuable tips save you 90% on the cost of yogurt, along with tasty ways of serving yogurt as pudding or chocolate pie. There are tips on saving 75% of the normal preparation time in cooking beans and whole grains, how to eat garlic bulbs that taste more like roasted nuts, how to make a healthy pizza, and even recipes for baking delicious and nutritious cookies and cakes.

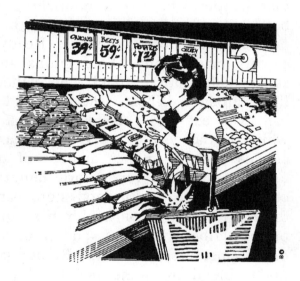

You can feed your body the nutrients it needs, plus save time in the kitchen, plus save about $1500 per year per family, plus derive great pleasure from eating by following these time tested recipes in my new book.

-animals & nutrition

NW of Tahlequah. My grandpa was a horse doctor long ago. He used to tell me that if the animal got sick they would first check the animals diet for clues on the problem. Why doesn't my doctor do that when I get sick?

Good question NW. The American Medical system is built around drugs and surgery, which can be very essential tools for certain emergency medical situations. However, these tools cannot correct the underlying causes in many degenerative diseases, such as heart disease, cancer, diabetes, arthritis and others. The old time physician and veterinarian had few therapeutic tools to work with and hence relied heavily on nutrition and herb therapy. Modern medicine lost interest in these therapies with the advent of antibiotics, laser surgery and other exciting developments in medical science. In order to have the world's best, most cost effective and clinically effective health care system, what we need is a balance of both the emergency medicine of drugs and surgery coupled with good old horse doctor sense that your grandpa had in using gentle healers of nutrients, herbs, and other modalities. Until then, we are just playing with half a deck.

-improving digestion

KP of Enid. I get this fullness after every meal that doesn't let up for a couple hours. I don't think that I'm overeating. What's the problem?

Thanks KP. You could be experiencing a common problem that sets in with maturity. Many of us gradually lose the ability to make enough hydrochloric acid and enzymes for proper digestion of our foods. When that happens, the food sits in the stomach for longer than normal and can ferment, like grains in an old moonshiners still. If you have fullness, or bloating, or considerable gas; then you may want to consider taking supplemental betaine hydrochloride or pancreatic enzymes, found in health food stores. These supplements are merely replacing what your body is no longer making in adequate quantities. If you find relief with these gentle natural substances, then your problem is solved. If your problem persists, then see your doctor.

-wet tissue paper for hemorrhoids

JT of Muskogee. I doubt that you will answer this one on the air, but I have a painful and nagging problem with hemorrhoids, that doesn't go away, even with ointments. Your help would be greatly appreciated.

You're right JT. I normally would not talk about hemorrhoids on the air, unless there were so many people like you are suffering unnecessarily. Did you know that the most commonly shoplifted item in American pharmacies is Preparation H, which gives you an idea of how common your problem is. Hemorrhoids are inflamed tissue near the anus, generally caused by abrasion or poor wound healing ability. The sphincter muscle in the rectum is a delicate tissue. It can be irritated by the passage of hard feces, which is a result of not enough fiber or fluid in the diet. Low intake of vitamin C can make the tissue slow to repair itself. Many pregnant women get hemorrhoids as the baby within is taking what little vitamin C is in the blood stream. Dry tissue paper can cause the problem, also. The solution is simple. Eat more fruit and vegetables and drink more water to soften the stools. Take supplements of magnesium, folacin, vitamin C, and Perfect 7 to improve the muscular contractions that push the feces through the system. And, listen up, wet your tissue paper before cleaning yourself after going to the bathroom. Just keep a cup of water by the toilet and cleanse yourself with wet paper, then softly dab it dry.

-husband now takes vitamins and continues to smoke

WB of Oklahoma City. My husband has finally agreed to start taking vitamins with the rest of the family, but he still continues to smoke and won't walk with us after dinner. Are the vitamins doing any good?

Thanks WB. Another concerned wife trying to keep her husband healthy. Guys, why is it that the scientific, logical, and Scripturally-based message of nutrition is better received by women than men? Back to you WB. All lifestyle factors are vectors, which are forces with both a specific strength and direction. For instance, person flying a small plane at 100 mph into a head wind of 120 mph has a ground speed of -20 mph. Similarly, a person who is taking vitamins, but not getting exercise and continuing to smoke has a negative ground speed, even though they are doing something right. In order to properly maintain this body, this temple of the soul, we need to get all our lifestyle vectors pushing the plane in the right direction. While taking vitamins can help some, it won't be nearly as helpful as long as your husband is continuing his destructive lifestyle practices, which are like flying a plane into a strong headwind.

-kids and vitamin supplements

CM of Sand Springs. My doctor says that my kids don't need to take vitamins as long as they eat right. Yet your books say otherwise.

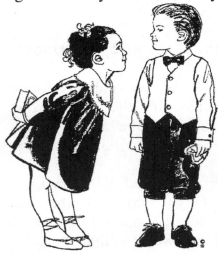

Thanks CM. While your doctor is providing information that used to be widely spread, it may not be accurate in light of new evidence. First of all, most kids do not eat right. We are all exposed to an endless array of nutrient-depleted junk food. If you watch the commercials that saturate the Saturday morning cartoons, then you know how easily swayed kids can be in eating junk food. Secondly, kids are growing rapidly. In order for growth to be ideal, it may require more nutrients than can be obtained from even a very good diet. Many kids are borderline anemic, even if they are eating good foods. Thirdly, there is a growing body of data that supports the difference between nutritional surviving and thriving. A study in England found that kids who took vitamin supplements had better

test scores than kids not taking vitamins. The
human brain grows rapidly through about age 7,
then stops. For better or for worse, the brain is
built from nutrients provided in the diet and
guided by the genetic blueprints inherited from a
child's parents. And fourth, many American
children already have the beginnings of heart
disease, which can be promoted through poor diet.
The new evidence says that every child should take
a good broad spectrum vitamin mineral supplement
to improve their health.

-change husband's eating habits
AD of Skiatook. My husband is a real creature
of habit and his habits aren't too healthy. But he
has agreed to make one simple change to improve
his diet. If I only have one shot at improving his
diet and he won't tolerate much change, what
should I do?
Tough question AD. There are many
guidelines that would improve the nutritional value
of the average American diet: such as eating less
fat, more fiber, more fruits and vegetables, using
whole grains rather than white flour, less soda pop
and sugary snack foods. But since you have to
make one simple change that will have a major
impact and he won't notice, I would recommend
serving him daily portions of carrot and cabbage
cole slaw. There is abundant evidence on the
therapeutic value of beta-carotene in carrots and
indoles in cabbage. A dozen major research centers
are pursuing this area. Grate up cabbage as you
would for cole slaw, then soak it overnight in a

mixture of vinegar and water. Next morning, drain the grated cabbage, add equal parts of grated carrots along with a small amount of Italian dressing with a sprinkling of sugar. Mix thoroughly. The vinegar soaking takes away the gas forming ability of cabbage. Scientists estimate that if every American would add 2 carrots and some cabbage to their diet, we could cut cancer incidence by 300,000 new cases per year.

-PAP smear came back positive

NL of Wagoner. My PAP smear came back with some bad news. My doctor says that I have stage 2 cervical dysplasia and that he may need to operate if it gets worse. I'm young and would like more children. Is there something I can do?

Yes, NL. Cervical dysplasia is abnormal growth on the cervix, near a woman's uterus. It can lead to cancer, which would require surgical remove of your organs, and no more kids. There is convincing evidence showing that the early stages of abnormal growth can be reversed with nutrients. Researchers at the University of Alabama and elsewhere have found that 10 mg of folacin coupled with 1 gram of vitamin C and 25,000 iu of beta carotene can reverse cervical dysplasia in the majority of women tested. Keep working with your doctor. If your condition gets worse, then you may need surgery. If you follow my advice and the information contained in my new book, BEATING CANCER WITH NUTRITION, then your condition will probably clear up.

Chapter 7

📖

HEALTH TIPS

☞ "Natural forces within us are the true healers."
Hippocrates, father of modern medicine, 400 BC

(opening) This is health tips and I'm Dr. Patrick
Quillin. Today's question comes from___
(closing) God Bless and good health.

-gut bacteria, yogurt & yeast infections

RK. I no sooner get off one batch of
medication for my vaginal yeast infection, than
another infection comes along. The drugs create
problems with my intestines. Is there some better
way to deal with a woman's yeast infections?

Most definitely. Yeast grows under the
favorable conditions of heat, moisture, and
darkness; which is why the vaginal tract of women
is more vulnerable than men's anatomy. However,
the immune system is also a critical link in beating
yeast problems. In various studies, women who
consume active cultured yogurt were able to
dramatically cut down on yeast infections. In one
study, the women on the yogurt experienced such
benefits that they were unwilling to give up their

yogurt to complete the cross over phase of the study. The bacteria in active yogurt competes with yeast to make conditions less favorable for yeast growth. God has blessed us with simple solutions for nearly every problem on earth.

-Epsom salts for spasms

BT. After decades of no exercise and an office job, I am finally trying to start a fitness program. However, I find that I sometimes get these heart problems that my doctor calls arhythmias. Any solutions from God's pharmacy?

God pharmacy--that's a good way of putting it! Work with your doctor to make sure that any possible dangerous heart problems are under medical supervision. Meanwhile, studies show that about 90% of heart attack patients are suffering from low magnesium levels. Magnesium helps in the relaxation phase of heart contractions. Low magnesium can surface as palpitations in the heart or spasms in muscles elsewhere in the body. Best food sources of magnesium are whole grains, dark green leafy vegetables, soybeans, molasses, peas, and liver. A simple supplement is to take a half teaspoon of food grade Epsom salts daily. Magnesium: the miracle mineral that most meals are missing.

-breast cancer, Tamoxifen & cabbage

NL. Since my mother and 2 aunts have all suffered with breast cancer, my doctor wants to either put me on Tamoxifen for life or do preventive surgery and remove my healthy breasts. Is this a good idea?

Thanks NL. While breast cancer now strikes one in nine American women, it is not in God's plan. American women are exposed to pollutants, stress, high fat diet, not enough fresh fruits and vegetables, and too much sugar--all of which elevates the risk for breast cancer. Tamoxifen may help in the short term, but if used too long it presents a cancer risk itself. Better to follow a strict cancer prevention program, such as outlined in my book BEATING CANCER WITH NUTRITION or CANCER AND NUTRITION by Dr. Charles Simone. Potent natural agents, like cabbage, fish oil, and vitamin C, can effectively shut down the cancer-causing ability of estrogen without the risky side effects of long term tamoxifen use.

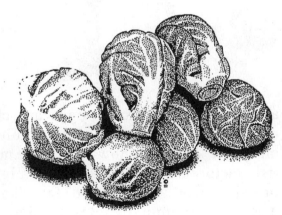

-eggs & heart disease

AH. You nutritionists ought to get your act together. One says don't eat eggs and another says eggs are okay. No wonder Americans are so confused about nutrition that they eat anything they want.

Thanks for your candor AH. For various reasons, nutrition has become almost as controversial as politics--but it shouldn't be. There are some very solid logical principles upon which the science of nutrition rests. Eggs, for instance, are one of the most basic of human foods. Eggs are

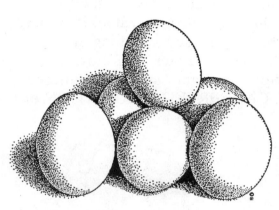 loaded with the best available protein, plus decent amounts of vitamin A and lecithin. The cholesterol in eggs has minimal impact on the serum cholesterol levels of 90% of humans, according to research. Eggs are cheap and are easy to chew and digest for older adults. Latest studies on heart disease show that the most predictable risk factor is low levels of vitamin E in the blood-- in other words, its rusted fats that cause heart disease. Vitamin E helps to slow down that rusting process. For most people, eggs are good food and for everyone, nutrition makes good sense.

-back problems & solutions

DP. My doctor says that the next step in treating my back problems may be surgery, but I'm not interested. Help with options, please.

Indeed, you are not alone. Up to 90% of adults suffer from back problems at some time in

their lives.   Problems are caused by poor posture,
no muscle development surrounding the spine,
sitting all day, stress, and injury.   Solutions include
exercises, getting relief from the pressure of
gravity, better posture, proper posture in lifting
objects, and therapy from chiropractors or
osteopaths.   A recent study in the New England
Journal of Medicine showed that millions of
Americans find relief from back problems through
chiropractic therapy.   Keep in mind that 80% of the
support for your spinal column comes from the
surrounding muscles.   If you have no muscles--then
there is no support for the critical spinal vertebrae,
which leads to problems.   Also, the use of hanging
bars, inversion swings, or back arches all can help
with back problems.   Surgery should be a last
resort option.

-tonsillitis & allergies

CT.   All three of my kids suffer from large
tonsils.   The doctor says that the easiest solution is
to have the tonsils taken out.   But it doesn't seem
like God would make us with optional body parts.

Thanks CT.   You are right.   There is a purpose
to all parts of this Divinely created human body.
Tonsils are filtering stations for the lymph system.
When the tonsils are enlarged, there is usually a
problem with the lymph system, either as an
allergy, or chronic infection, or toxic burden.   Likely
suspects for allergies include milk, wheat, or beef.
A weak immune system can be recharged with
nutrients like vitamin A, E, C, B-6, zinc, and
selenium.   Or detoxification of the body may be

necessary with large amounts of fiber, clean water, and herbal purgatives like Perfect 7. If the immune system is working properly and if allergies can be controlled, then the tonsils will return to their normal function.

-link between mental health & physical health

ZL. Since the loss of Mom, I can see my Dad just dying before our eyes. What can we do?

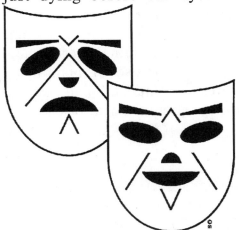

In Proverbs we read "A merry doeth good, but a broken spirit dries up the bones." Philosophers and religious leaders have told us for centuries about the link between the mind and body. We now find concrete scientific evidence that links the chemicals produced in the mind with immediate effects on the body. For instance, according to years of research, the most predictable risk factor in heart disease is loneliness. Dr. Candace Pert of the National Institutes of Health has found that the mind is a "pharmacy" and is on duty 24 hours a day, making substances that will either improve or worsen health. Jesus told us to "Rejoice, and again I say rejoice". In today's heavily polluted society with stress taking its toll on people, those words become ever so valuable. Unless your Dad can find a rebirth of spirit on his own or with counselling help, his broken spirit may well lead to his physical downfall.

-hot dogs and cancer

VM. I've got two kids ages 3 and 6 who live on hot dogs. That's obviously not the best food, but is it okay for awhile?

Maybe not. In two large studies, researchers found that intake of processed meats, specifically hot dogs and bologna were linked to a higher risk for leukemia in children and brain cancer if mother consumed processed meats while pregnant. Hot dogs have a number of nutritional question marks: 1) They are high in fat, which is about 2/3 of the calories, 2) Since most pollutants are fat soluble, that high fat content carries with it more pollutants, 3) and finally sodium nitrite is a coloring agent and preservative that carries some cancer risk. Also, we find that bad diets are a double edged sword. That is, you have problems in what you are eating and you do not get protection from foods that you should be

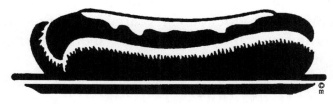

eating; such as whole grains, beans, fruits and vegetables. Hot dogs and bologna might be okay once a week, but I would not encourage these foods as a staple in the diet.

-phytochemicals in plants

JR.   An article in Newsweek magazine talked about phytochemicals as being even more important than vitamins.   Do you agree?

Phytochemicals are substances found in plants (hence the term phyto) that have potent abilities to improve our health.   Researchers are astounded by the sheer number of phytochemicals, which is well beyond 20,000 at this point. Lycopenes in tomatoes help to stop the effects of disease and aging.   Allicin in garlic is so effective at lowering blood fats and pressure that it outperforms many expensive drugs.   Indole 3 carbinol in cabbage helps to detoxify the body and escort estrogen out before it can trigger cancer. Genistein in soybeans may well become a potent agent in the war on cancer.   In Genesis, we read, "Behold I have given you every plant and it shall be food for you." On any given fall day, you can see the red, orange, yellow, and purple pigments in autumn foliage that make up some of these phytochemicals. While phytochemicals are not more important than vitamins, they surely will merit their own chapter in upcoming nutrition books.

-anti-oxidants

TC.   After years of listening to my doctor bad mouth vitamins, he is now coming around to recommending some anti-oxidants for my husband's heart disease.   I still don't understand what an anti-oxidant or free radical is.

Put simply, free radicals are the bad guys because they are electron thieves. If they steal an electron from the DNA blueprints, or the vital cell membrane, then free radicals make that molecule into something that is unstable, which could lead to cancer, premature aging, or one of many degenerative diseases like cataracts. Antioxidants are the good guys, like vitamins C, E, and beta-carotene. These substances are electron donors. Instead of allowing the bad guys to destroy your own tissue, these antioxidants give up an electron, like a sacrificial lamb, to spare your tissue from destruction. Almost all antioxidants are found in plant food and account for the fact that 200 studies have now shown that a diet rich in fruits and vegetables will lower the risk for most common diseases in America.

-brown fatty tissue & weight loss

LF. My weight problems seem to get worse with each diet that I try. What am I going to do?

Actually, dieting may be bad for you. Researchers now find that withholding food and calories can cause a number of problems. 1) Your body looks for protein to fill a critical need and may eat away at your vital organs, like the heart. 2) When you eat nothing for long periods, you send signals to your body that food intake is unpredictable and therefore the body should become very stingy with the fat calories that are stored. Thyroid function can be lowered, which then makes the body an incredibly efficient machine at storing calories. This whole process can be reversed through eating less fat, eating small frequent meals, regular exercise, and jump starting your body's heat furnace in a process called thermogenesis. MaHuang, caffeine, hydroxycitrate, and aspirin have been shown to help trigger the body's brown fat into burning excess calories for heat. There is plenty of reasons for hope in your situation.

-herbal tranquilizer

AR. I have been through a rough stretch with my recent divorce and loss of my sister. I do rely on prayer and don't want to get hooked on sedative drugs, but sure could use some mild natural tranquilizing agent?

You are taking the right approach to grief and stress. There are some herbs that have been demonstrated in scientific studies to have the same or better tranquilizing effect as prescription drugs, yet do not have the side effects, cost, or habit-forming problems. Kava-kava, valerian, and ginseng have all passed scientific scrutiny as providing tranquilizing relief in human studies. Also, let your emotions be expressed through tears, talking, and writing out your feelings. Exercise can be an excellent stress reliever. God has given us the tools to cope with any problem in life. The grieving process takes time. Remember, a diamond is nothing more than a piece of coal that was put under extreme pressure.

-licorice & ulcers

RM. My ulcers aren't getting any better with medication. My doctor says that surgery may be the next option.

As long as surgery is the last option. New scientific evidence shows that ulcers can be triggered by a bacteria. Which means that anti- biotics have found new favor in treating some types of ulcers. Also, a clinical trial using the herb licorice found it to be superior to the preferred drug, Tagamet, in treating ulcers. When 874 ulcer patients were given either Tagamet or the active form of licorice, deglycyrrhizinated licorice, for 6 weeks, licorice provided improvement for 77% vs 63% for Tagament. Remember, the licorice candy you buy has no active licorice herb in it, but rather synthetic flavoring agents. Once again, God's pharmacy is superior.

-smoking & lobelia

BK. I have tried to beat my smoking habit and just can't do it. I know its not good for me, but I started smoking long ago, when all the movie stars were doing it. Now I'm hooked and need help.

You and millions of other Americans suffer from an addiction that is 6 times more powerful than crack cocaine: tobacco. One fourth of Americans still smoke and most of these people will suffer needlessly and die prematurely from this lethal drug. Studies show that most smokers start in their teens and get hooked. Kicking the habit usually requires an iron will, plus some behavioral counselling such as found in seminars and audiotape series, plus the herb lobelia to reduce the cravings for smoking. Most health authorities agree that the single greatest risk factor in American health is smoking. You can beat it.

-controlling blood sugar

DJ. Your book, BEATING CANCER WITH NUTRITION, speaks of cancer being a sugar-feeder. But I thought that bread and potatoes eventually end up as sugar in the blood. I'm confused.

Very perceptive, DJ. Yes, all carbohydrate food, including squash, beans, bread, grains, and vegetables, will eventually end up being absorbed as glucose and fructose sugar into the blood. The issue at stake is "glycemic index" or how much sugar is found in the blood at any given time. Too little sugar will send the patient into the weakness, muscle tremors, and depression of hypoglycemia. Too much sugar in the blood will trigger diabetic coma, or the many complications of diabetes, or accelerate cancer growth, while also changing prostaglandins toward an unhealthy direction. Controlling blood sugar is a crucial focal point of health. Eat no white sugar. Only eat sweet foods, like fruit and honey, with a mixed meal, which helps to slow down rises in blood glucose. Eat complex carbohydrates like vegetables, grains and legumes. Get enough chromium, zinc, and B-6 to allow your body to process sugar and insulin. You can make optimal blood sugar levels your vehicle to better mental and physical energy levels.

-mercury fillings

FJ. I used to work in a factory that used mercury. We were told to be careful since mercury is a poison. So why does my dentist want to put mercury fillings in my daughter's teeth?

Good question. Mercury is a deadly poison and was first highlighted with the mad hatter found in Lewis Carroll's ALICE IN WONDERLAND. Mercury causes poisoning of the nervous system as well as interfering with energy metabolism which can affect the heart and every cell in the body. Silver fillings for dental cavities contain about 30% mercury. Eventually, all fillings erode over time and are 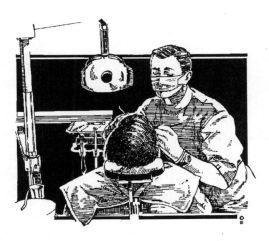 swallowed. Even fillings that are intact create a battery effect in the mouth, just like the battery in your car. With thousands of studies to support the notion that mercury is a poison, it doesn't make sense to put it in the mouth. In one Swedish study, mercury amalgams were replaced with composite fillings and that group experienced a 30% reduction in sick days for the coming year. If you avoid sugar and brush and floss the teeth regularly, then there may be no need for fillings. But if fillings are necessary, use composite fillings without mercury.

-impotence, heart disease & drugs

TN. My husband has been having a rough time in the last few years, with heart disease, bypass surgery, and drugs for his high blood pressure. Although it isn't important to me, he is further bothered by the impotence all this has created. Any help?

Yes. In a study of over 400 men with impotence, researchers found that 90% of these older men had advanced heart disease. When blood vessels are blocked with fatty deposits, such as occurs in coronary artery disease, some physicians will chose bypass surgery for relief. When blood pressure gets too high, most physicians will use drugs to help lower the pressure. Yet both heart disease, and the medication for high blood pressure can cause impotence. By cleaning out the arteries with natural agents like Hawthorne, chromium, niacin, fiber and a low fat diet, coupled with exercise and stress reduction; you can return the plugged up vessels to normal clear passage and improve sexual functions. By using natural agents to lower blood pressure, like magnesium, potassium, fish oil, and vitamin C, a person can be weaned of medication and help to restore natural sexual function.

Chapter 8

📖

HEALTH TIPS

☞ "The secret to success in life is to eat what you like and let the foods fight it out inside." Mark Twain, famous humorist

(opening) This is Health Tips and I'm Dr. Patrick Quillin. Today's question comes from ___
(closing) God Bless and good health.

-Ancestral diet
VN. In your book, HEALING SECRETS FROM THE BIBLE, you mention the need to eat closer to Abraham's diet. What does that have to do with my health problems?

Quite simply, God built the magnificent human body and God created our elegantly nourishing food supply. When we heavily spray our crops with poisons, then slice, dice, chop, blend and hydrogenate God's food, then add 2800 different FDA approved food additives, we have seriously curtailed the healing power of the food. When we live on stress, toxins, tobacco, alcohol, drugs and not enough rest and prayer, we reduce the body's ability to live a long and healthy life. In

Abraham's day, nearly 4000 years ago, our ancestors ate a pure diet of unprocessed foods and often lived a vigorous life of 120 years, like Moses.

-90 and 10 rule

TA. To be honest, I just can't seem to resist a desert now and again. Is that bad for me?

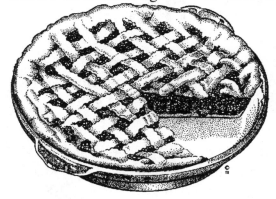

No. If you are healthy, then I recommend the 90/10 rule: on any given day, let 90% of your food intake be healthy and nourishing, while the remaining 10% is unimportant and can be spent on less nourishing foods. This ratio allows for realistic eating in modern America, for eating out with friends, or on airplanes, or an occasional pizza at an office party. This means that a small desert or fast food meal once in awhile is okay, but should not become the general rule. If you are at your Grandma's for her 80th birthday party, have some of the cake she baked. It will be good for you.

-why did I get cancer

LK. I feel like I have been cheated. I always ate right and didn't smoke, but I came down with the cancer last year.

I understand your frustration. Most diseases involve a long list of risk factors. With cancer, the risk factors include: diet, exercise, attitude, toxins, and genetics. Beyond the obvious voluntary toxins of drugs, alcohol, and tobacco, there are many toxins that enter our food, air, and water supply, which has increased the incidence of cancer in Americans. We dump 1.2 billion pounds of pesticides on our crops annually, add 4 million pounds of antibiotics to cows and chickens to help them grow faster, dump 90 billion pounds of toxic waste into our 55,000 toxic waste sites across this fair land. 50 million Americans breath air that is unhealthy while 40% of our fresh water supply has been rendered unfit for drinking. Because of these violation of God's green earth, we have a cancer epidemic on our hands, sometimes in people like you who make efforts to live a healthy life. Though only 1 out of a thousand of our ancient ancestors might develop cancer, today 1 out of 3 Americans will get this disease. We need to clean up our air, food, and water supply while improving nutrient intake and stress levels before we will get this cancer epidemic under control.

-catfish

MP. Is catfish OK to eat?

In small amounts, yes. The reason catfish is so popular is because it is high in fat, which creates a problem for people with a tendency toward heart disease and obesity. Also, catfish is usually breaded and deep fried, which further adds to the empty calories and fat content. Also, catfish caught in polluted rivers and lakes would have high amounts of toxins in the meat. Most catfish, fortunately, is raised on catfish farms where the pollution level is under control. There is evidence now that only 2 servings of fish per week can cut the risk for heart attack in half. In order to get more of the healthy fat, called omega 3 fats, better fish choices than catfish would include salmon, tuna, swordfish, halibut, and bass. Fish in general is a healthy food, and catfish eaten sparingly can be a welcome addition to the diet of a healthy person.

-rewards for lifestyle changes

PD. I want to make some serious improvements in my diet and exercise program, but I don't know how to encourage myself without the reward of food.

Very good point. At our very core, humans all operate on the simple principle that we want to move away from discomfort and toward pleasure. When changing the diet and exercising means moving toward discomfort and away from pleasure, the program is doomed to failure. We have to make it fun, and we have to reward ourselves for accomplishments. For instance, set realistic goals of losing 1 pound per week for the next 12 weeks. As you achieve this goal, put a gold star on the calendar each week in your kitchen. When you exercise, put a silver star on your calendar for that day. When you have avoided an unhealthy temptation of snack food, give yourself another star. Reward yourself with a music tape, or dress, or shoes, or promise yourself a hot bubble bath. If you can offer yourself enough incentive and make

lifestyle changes fun, then you will make it a
lifetime achievement.

**-exercise vs. tamoxifen in preventing breast
cancer**

KQ. My sister has become part of a study to
see if tamoxifen will reduce breast cancer incidence.
Since several members of my family had breast
cancer, should I take tamoxifen also?

Only you and your doctor can make that
decision. But let me provide you with some
information to help you make a wise choice.
Tamoxifen can slow down and possibly prevent
certain types of breast
cancer. Yet when taken
long term tamoxifen
increases the risk for
cervical and liver cancer
as well as eye damage.
While studies show that
30 minutes daily of
exercise reduces the risk
for breast cancer by 75%
with a long list of
beneficial side effects,
the best hope for
tamoxifen is to reduce
breast cancer incidence
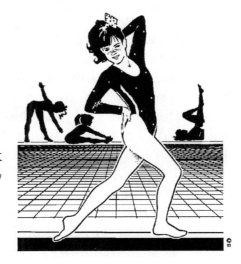
by 20%. There are safer and more natural ways to
avoid breast cancer, by stimulating your God-given
healing forces within your body.

-how to work brown rice into the diet

CT. My kids won't eat brown rice, telling me that it looks dirty. How can I slip it past them?

Americans need more fiber in the diet, and whole grains, like brown rice are a good way to boost the fiber intake. Dr. John Kellogg started the cereal empire in the 19th century by simple adding bran fiber to a nation of constipated people. To help infiltrate your recipes with whole grains, try mixing your white rice with brown rice in increasingly higher ratios. In the beginning, start off with 7 parts white rice and 1 part brown rice, thoroughly mixed together. Next week, use 6 parts white rice with 1 part brown rice, and so on. You can do the same thing with cooking cakes and muffins. Start slowly adding whole grain flour, such as wheat, rye, buckwheat, oats, and barley to your normal white flour recipes. Remember to add extra fluid to allow for the absorbant properties of the fiber. By the time you reach 75-100% whole grain flour, no one will have noticed the change and there will be a new found level of health in your home.

-alcohol cravings

BV. I am a saved Christian but I still crave alcohol. Any suggestions?

Yes. Alcoholism can be caused by a number of physical and psychological factors. For instance, combat veterans are more likely to become alcoholics, which means that these people need to heal the spiritual hurt from such a harsh experience. There are also physical solutions to the alcohol cravings that many people have. Stabilize blood sugar levels through avoidance of white sugar and caffeine, eat small frequent meals, exercise, take supplements of chromium, B-6, and the oils from flax or fish. Some alcoholics get great relief by using supplements of glutamine. One of the more productive scientists of this century, Dr. Roger Williams, wrote a book on Nutrition and Alcoholism which should be read by everyone with a drug or alcohol problem. There are oftentimes simples solutions for complex modern health problems.

-leg cramps at night

WR. What can I do about cramps in my feet at night?

There are a number of simple remedies that can cure this problem. The nutrients magnesium, potassium, and calcium are often missing in the diets of people with leg cramps. Supplements of these minerals plus vitamin E can help. Make sure that your feet are not tucked in too tightly under the sheets, so that the calf muscles are constantly tensed. Take a tablespoon of raw unpasteurized apple cider vinegar in 4 ounces of apple cider at bedtime. Leg cramps can be caused by circulation problems, which involves lowering fat in the diet and using vitamin C, E, chromium, fish oil, and lecithin to help clear out the clogged blood vessels. Leg cramps are a common but easily treated problem.

-don't want to use antibiotics

JT. My children are in that age range where they are constantly getting infections. I don't want to use antibiotics too often. What are some natural substitutes?

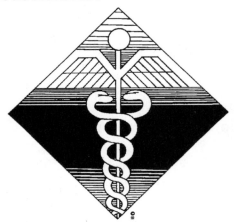

You are right to be concerned about the overuse of antibiotics, which are only for bacterial infections like staphylococcus, not for viral infections like the flu or Chronic Fatigue Syndrome. Excess antibiotic use has led to the development of super germs which are resistant to the strongest antibiotics available. Some natural alternatives as listed in my book, HEALING SECRETS FROM THE BIBLE, include: colloidal silver, garlic, echinecea, golden seal, licorice, beta-carotene, vitamin C, zinc lozenges, bovine cartilage, aloe vera, and vitamin E. What these natural substances do is bolster the quantity and quality of immune factors that protect us against infections, aging, and cancer. God's pharmacy was here long before man's pharmacy, and usually includes safer and cheaper options than drugs.

-soda pop

NK. Is it bad for my kids to drink a lot of soda pop?

Yes. Soft drinks are basically lots of water, of questionable purity, with lots of sugar, caffeine, phosphoric acid, and chemicals that offer color and flavor. If we could only see the Coca-Cola exhibit in Atlanta, which shows that if the Old Faithful geyser in Yellowstone Park would gush Coca cola for 1500 years, it would never catch up with the volume of soft drinks consumed around the world. Diet soft drinks may be even more harmful than regular sugar soft drinks. Aspartame or Nutrasweet and saccharin or Equal have serious side effects. There is growing evidence that sensitive individuals who consume Nutrasweet develop everything from memory loss, to labored breathing to even more serious nervous disorders. Instead of soft drinks, substitute dilute fruit juices with vitamin C, or iced tea, or apple cider with a sprinkling of cider vinegar, or purified water, or ginger tea.

-why do we get sick?

RS. I work as a nurse and see a lot of sick people, do you think God wants us to be ill?

No. John 3:16 begins "for God so loved the world". We read in Luke "your Father is pleased to give you the kingdom". Based upon many references in Scripture and the beauty that God has created all around us, we can be confident that God wants us to be healthy. Yet with every gift there is a condition. Most of our health problems are self-inflicted, as I outline in my book, HEALING SECRETS FROM THE BIBLE. We cause the problem, not God. When Mr. Jones commented on what a fine garden that God had produced for his wife, she replied "Yes, but you should have seen it before I got here." The take home lesson is clear: God will work wondrous miracles in all of us all day every day, but we have to put forth some effort, just as we do with a garden. God wants us to be well, and we have to become active participants in the process. Hosea 4:9 says: My people perish from lack of knowledge.

-sugar & kid's behavior

AD. My kids come home from the grandparents wild eyed with all the sugar they eat. What can I tell my folks to serve my kids so that everyone is happy?

Grandparents often want to show their love to the grandkids through food. As long as that food helps to build a strong mind and body, this is a good kind of spoiling. Ask your folks to try a breakfast of whole wheat English muffins with a mixture of cinnamon, butter and honey on top. Cinnamon is a potent herb for improving insulin action and blood glucose regulation. The whole wheat bread with higher fiber content will also slow down the absorption of sugar into the blood stream. Make pancakes with 2 eggs and a banana blended in with 1/2 cup of oat or buckwheat flour. You can satisfy the sweet tooth of a child, and the needs of a grandparent without sacrificing the health needs of the child and the mental health of the parents.

-meat & the Bible

ER. What does the Bible say about eating meat

Prior to the flood, Noah's people were vegetarians, or did not eat animal products. After the flood, God gave His people permission to eat certain fish, poultry, beef, and lamb. While the argument about vegetarianism is loaded with ethics and emotions, the human body is built to tolerate and sometimes even require a certain amount of animal tissue. Eskimos consume 60% of their calories from high fat fish and have

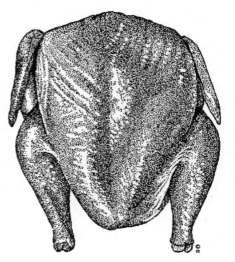

virtually no cancer or heart disease to speak of. Meanwhile, there is clear evidence that most people would be healthier eating little or no animal tissue and the earth could support a lot more people, since we get about 20 times more protein from an acre of soy versus an acre used to grow beef. If you eat meat, then chose small amounts of creatures that run, swim, or fly, meaning active creatures. One third of your meal plate should include low fat high protein food, such as turkey, chicken, fish, and beans.   One third of the plate should come from unprocessed and uncooked plant food, such as fresh fruit and green leafy vegetables.   The remaining one third of the diet should come from unprocessed but cooked plant food, like wheat, oats, beans, yams, and cauliflower.

-organic   produce

LR.   I can't get organic produce year round, what are the options

Grow your own is best, followed by organic produce, followed by fresh locally grown produce in season.   Next best is fresh produce from your grocery store that has been either peeled or soaked in warm water with vinegar to remove the pesticide residues.   The National Academy of Sciences has estimated that about 1% of all cancer in this country, or 16,000 people each year, get cancer from pesticide residues on the food supply. Many pesticides can lower the immune system, damage the DNA, and affect the brain.   As explained in my book HEALING SECRETS FROM THE BIBLE, you can inexpensively grow your own sprouts in your kitchen for fresh produce year round without any chemical sprays.   It is important to keep your food supply as clean as is possible.

-recipes in the Bible?

TL.   Are there any recipes in the Bible

Actually, yes.   In Ezekial 4:9 we read: "take wheat and barley, beans and lentils, millet and

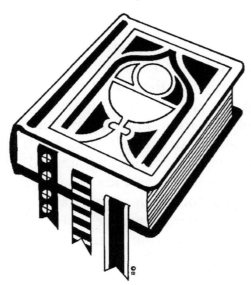

spelt, put them in a storage jar and use them to make bread for yourself."   Only in the past few decades have scientists become aware of the need to match plant foods in order to get high quality protein while on a vegetarian diet.   This Scripture verse tells us to match the whole grains of wheat, millet, spelt, and barley with the legumes of beans and lentils, then sprout them to increase bioavailability of nutrients for a resulting delicious bread.   This Ezekial bread is available at most grocery stores.   This is just another example where you can find the wisdom of the ages along with good science in God's cookbook for a good life, the Bible.

-malnutrition in spite of plenty of food

BW.   How can there be malnutrition in America, when we pay our farmers not to grow crops?

Good question. Oddly enough, Howard Hughes, the multi-billionaire, died of malnutrition. Americans have no problems with quantity of food, but we are making poor choices at the dinner table. We grow enough food in this country to get half of us overweight, to throw away enough food to feed an additional 50 million people each day, and to ship enough food overseas to somewhat offset our trade imbalance. Yet in spite of our enviable volume of food that is available, the quality of our diet is quite poor, as we eat too much of the wrong things and not enough of the right things. Based upon major government surveys, we eat too much fat, salt, sugar, food additives, alcohol, and animal food, while not getting enough of various vitamins, minerals, fiber, complex carbohydrates, special fats in fish and flax, and clean water. In many countries and for much of history, malnutrition meant not enough food. In America, malnutrition means not using good judgment in food selection. The land of plentiful harvest is also a land where many of our health problems are caused by malnutrition.

-detoxification

CM. what does the Bible have to say about toxins and detoxification

Paul tells us in 2 Corinthians 7:1 "let us purify ourselves of everything that contaminates body and spirit". Somewhere between the voluntary poisons of drugs, alcohol, and tobacco, along with the involuntary poisons that permeate our food, air, and water supply, Americans have developed many diseases from toxic burden. Detoxification involves eliminating these unwanted poisons through the avenues of urine, feces, sweat, and liver, as outlined in my book, HEALING SECRETS FROM THE BIBLE. Increase your intake of clean water, fiber, vitamin C, selenium, herbs like psyllium and cascara sagrada. Allow the body to detoxify through sweating from exercise and hot tubs. Some people include fasting, chelation, and enemas as more aggressive approaches to detoxification, which has become crucial for the healing of many Americans.

-need some energy

SA. My get up and go got up and went with the birth of my 4th child, I need energy help big time.

Take a high dose B-complex supplement first thing in the morning along with some lecithin in your cereal or yogurt. Make sure that you get adequate sleep. Ironically, when you are tired, you may be in need of some exercise to thoroughly oxygenate your brain and body. There are herbs that can provide significant energy boosts, including guarana, gotu kola, ginseng, ma huang, and hot brewed tea. Many people are tired because of a toxic burden, which means that you may need to detoxify, as outlined in my book, HEALING SECRETS FROM THE BIBLE. Since you mentioned your 4th child, you may also be suffering from a hormonal imbalance, which can be helped by DHEA, or progesterone topically applied to the thigh region, or the herb diascorea or wild Mexican yam. Also, pace yourself. Too many women today have unrealistic expectations of themselves. Take time to nurture yourself, or you won't have the energy to nurture others.

-thermogenics and fat loss

KR. What is thermogenics and how can it help with my weight problem?

Thermogenics is the process of making heat from stored fat calories. We all have a certain amount of brown adipose tissue which wants to squander fat in a heat making process, with the net effect of keeping us warm and lean. Yet, through stress, malnutrition, toxic burden, sedentary lifestyle, and bundling up too much, we shut down this vital thermogenic process, which is partly responsible for our high incidence of obesity in America. To get your thermogenic mechanisms running again, regularly add garlic, hot peppers, ginger, horseradish, and cinnamon to your diet. Turn your home thermostat down to 65 in the winter and don't bundle up as much with warm clothing. Force your body to start generating some heat by burning that stored fat. Get some regular exercise. You can effortlessly melt away about 25 pounds of body fat in one year by gearing up your God-given thermogenic systems.

-forgiveness & healing

EK. Why would you mention forgiveness in your book HEALING SECRETS FROM THE BIBLE?

Of all the causes of disease in America, which include poor nutrition, stress, toxic burden, and no exercise, the most important of these factors is stress. The Bible is the first and best manual on healing emotional hurts. The greatest risk factor in heart disease is loneliness, or lack of love. Hate creates much social and health problems, too. Yet, Jesus taught us in the Our Father to "forgive us our debts as we forgive our debtors". Jesus told Peter to forgive your brother not seven but seventy seven times. Much mental and physical illness is brought about by the inability to forgive. Let it go. Get out the rage and emotions in a constructive fashion by beating on a pillow, crying, or writing out your feelings in a diary. Then let God cleanse your spirit. When we hate others, we only do ourselves harm, not the other person. Healing in body, mind, and spirit often times begins with forgiveness.

APPENDIX

☞ "And the earth brought forth vegetation, plants yielding seed after their kind and trees bearing fruit with seed in them after their kind. And God saw that it was good." Genesis 1:12

GOOD NUTRITION REFERENCES:

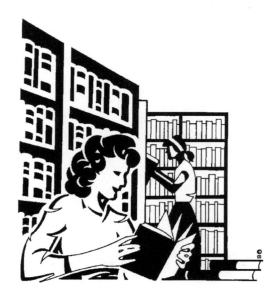

-Anderson, WELLNESS MEDICINE, Keats, 1987

-Balch & Balch, PRESCRIPTION FOR NUTRITIONAL HEALING, Avery, 1993

-Eaton, PALEOLITHIC PRESCRIPTION, Harper & Row, 1988

-Grabowski, RJ, CURRENT NUTRITIONAL THERAPY, Image Press, 1993

-Haas, STAYING HEALTHY WITH NUTRITION, Celestial, 1992

-Hausman, THE RIGHT DOSE, Rodale, 1987

-Hendler, DOCTOR'S VITAMIN AND MINERAL
ENCYCLOPEDIA, Simon & Schuster,1990
-Lieberman, S. et al., REAL VITAMIN & MINERAL
BOOK, Avery, 1990
-Murray, M, et al., ENCYCLOPEDIA OF NATURAL
MEDICINE, Prima, 1990
-National Research Council, RECOMMENDED DIETARY
ALLOWANCES, Nat Academy, 1989
-Price, NUTRITION AND PHYSICAL DEGENERATION,
Keats, 1989
-Quillin, P., HEALING NUTRIENTS, Random House,
1987
-Shils, ME, et al., MODERN NUTRITION IN HEALTH &
DISEASE, Lea & Febiger, 1994
-Werbach, M, NUTRITIONAL INFLUENCES ON
ILLNESS, Third Line, 1993

WHERE TO BUY NUTRITION PRODUCTS BY MAIL ORDER

BULK FOODS

Allergy Resources Inc., 195 Huntington Beach Dr.,
Colorado Springs, CO 80921, ph 719-488-3630
Deer Valley Farm, RD#1, Guilford, NY 13780, ph.
607-674-8556
Diamond K Enterprises, Jack Kranz, R.R. 1, Box 30, St.
Charles, MN 55972, ph. 507-932-4308
Gravelly Ridge Farms, Star Route 16, Elk Creek, CA
95939, ph. 916-963-3216
Green Earth, 2545 Prairie St., Evanston, IL 60201,
ph. 800-322-3662

Healthfoods Express, 181 Sylmar Clovis, CA 93612, ph. 209-252-8321

Jaffe Bros. Inc., PO Box 636, Valley Center, CA 92082, ph. 619-749-1133

Macrobiotic Wholesale Co., 799 Old Leicester Hwy, Asheville, NC 28806, ph. 704-252-1221

Moksha Natural Foods, 724 Palm Ave., Watsonville, CA, 95076, ph. 408-724-2009

Mountain Ark Co., 120 South East Ave., Fayetteville, AR, 72701, ph. 501-442-7191, or 800-643-8909

New American Food Co., PO Box 3206, Durham, NC 27705, ph. 919-682-9210

Timber Crest Farms, 4791 Dry Creek, Healdsburg, CA, 95448, ph. 707-433-8251, FAX -8255

Walnut Acres, Walnut Acres Road, Penns Creek, PA 17862, ph. 717-837-0601

LARGE STORES THAT SELL VITAMINS, MINERALS, & SOME HERBS BY MAIL

Bronson, 800-235-3200

NutriGuard, 800-433-2402

Health Center for Better Living, 813-566-2611

Vitamin Research Products, 800-877-2447

Vitamin Trader, 800-334-9310

Terrace International, 800-824-2434

Willner Chemists, 800-633-1106

STORES THAT SPECIALIZE IN SELLING HERBS BY MAIL

Gaia Herbals, 800-994-9355
Frontier Herbs 800-786-1388; fax 319-227-7966
Blessed Herbs 800-489-HERB; fax 508-882-3755
Trout Lake Farm 509-395-2025
San Francisco Herb Co. fax 800-227-5430
Star West 800-800-4372

RECOMMENDED COOKBOOKS

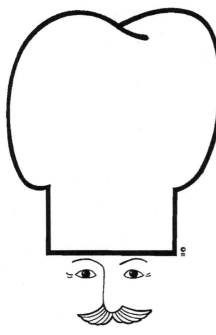

Kathy Cooks Naturally, Kathy Hoshijo
Super Seafood, Tom Ney
Eat Well, Live Well, Pamela Smith
Natural Foods Cookbook, Mary Estella
American Cancer Society Cookbook, Anne Lindsay
Mix & Match Cooking for Health, Jennie Shapter
The Healthy Gourmet Cookbook, Barbara Bassett
How to Use Natural Foods Deliciously, Barbara Bassett

The I Can't Believe This has No Sugar Cookbook,
Deborah Buhr
Eat Smart for a Healthy Heart Cookbook, Dr. Denton
Cooley & Dr. Carolyn Moore
Simply Light Cooking, Kitchens of Weight Watchers
Healthy Life-Style Cookbook, Weight Watchers
The American Health Food Book, Robert Barnett,
Nao Hauser
The Chez Eddy Living Heart Cookbook, Antonio
Gotto Jr.